Secrets of a Diabetic

A Natural Approach to Great Health

Gail Parker M.Ed

All information in Secrets of a Diabetic book is based on the experience, opinion and research of the author and of other healthcare professionals. This information is shared with the understanding that you accept full responsibility for your own health and well-being. We are all unique and the result and action of every remedy reflects as such. Health care covers a wide range of overall wellness; any suggestion herein cannot always be anticipated and never guaranteed. The author and publisher are not responsible for any adverse effects or consequences resulting from the use of any remedies, procedures, recipes, or preparations included in Secrets of a Diabetic book. Consult with your inner self, healthcare professionals, trained healers, and trusted friends in addition to the words written here.

Copyright © 2015 by Gail Parker, M.Ed.

All rights reserved. No part of this book may be reproduced or transmitted in any form or by any means without written permission from the author.

Printed and bound in the USA.

Edited by: TBL Business Solutions, LLC
Cover Design by: Krystina Taylor Parker, LLC

ISBN-13: 978-0692901120
ISBN-10: 0692901124
Library of Congress and Catalog: TXu 1-962-731

DEDICATION

This book is dedicated to:

My late grandmother, Stella. I wish I knew then what I know now, because I probably could have helped to extend your life.

My late grandfather, Archibald, for instilling self-discipline; you exemplified every aspect of a man. Thank you for loving me unconditionally.

My mother, June. Your life has taught me to continue pressing forward and never give up. Your life is a demonstration that nothing is given; it takes hard work and determination.

My husband, John. Your continuous love and support gives me encouragement to live a healthy lifestyle. You remind me that with constant incremental improvements, better health is possible.

My daughter, Krystina, you are a blessing. Your presence motivates me to be my best every day, and to be a role model for you and future generations.

I am thankful that you all influenced my life in some aspect. You make me want to be my best and live the best life possible.

TABLE OF CONTENTS

ABOUT THE AUTHOR 5
DISCLAIMER 7
Introduction: *Why you will love Secrets of a Diabetic - A Natural Approach to Great Health* 8
CHAPTER 1 *A "Trini" Girl* 27
CHAPTER 2 *What Is Your Gut Saying?* 43

Secret One: Be Calm - Your Life Depends On It
CHAPTER 3 *All About You* 59
CHAPTER 4 *Meditation* 77
CHAPTER 5 *Good Night* 93

Secret Two: Food for Life
CHAPTER 6 *"Toxic" Dinner* 107
CHAPTER 7 *The "Art" of Cooking* 117
CHAPTER 8 *God's Gracious Gift* 123

Secret Three: Eat to Lose - The Power of Food
CHAPTER 9 *Healthy Meals on a Dime - Weekly Planned Meals* 133
CHAPTER 10 *It's Never Too Late: EAT this, NOT this* 143
CHAPTER 11 *Got Milk?!?* 147
CHAPTER 12 *The Skinny on Carbs* 155

Secret Four: Get Movin' - Build Habits Not Equipment
CHAPTER 13 *On The Move* 169
CHAPTER 14 *Variety is the Spice of Life* 181
CHAPTER 15 *Healthy is the New Sexy* 193

Secret Five: Natural Healing
CHAPTER 16 *Natural Remedies - Herbs, Supplements, and Vitamins* 203
CHAPTER 17 *Herbs, Teas, and Essential Oils* 217
CHAPTER 18 *"Food As Thy Medicine"* 229
FINAL WORDS 239
RECIPES 251
BIBLIOGRAPHY 269

ABOUT THE AUTHOR
GAIL PARKER

LIFESTYLIST - Inspiring You To Build Healthy Habits

Visionary, Mentor, Speaker, Nutritional Advisor, Life Extender - these are just a few adjectives that describe Gail Parker. In her efforts to help you reach your highest self, Gail's personal walk with diabetes and other health concerns will encourage you to break unhealthy habits, and begin to defy diabetes and other health concerns naturally, even before it happens. Her knowledge and expertise will empower you; she will push you to the very edge of your comfort zone, where success truly begins. Gail's exhilarating and invigorating presence compels people to take back what has been stolen from them - health and a good quality of life. You will discover how to confront and deal with challenges that could hinder your progress toward living the lifestyle you most desire and deserve.

Gail has broad experience and a successful record of accomplishments in everything she touches. As a *Life Stylist*, she has worked with women and men of all ages for the last 25 years in what she believes is her mission in life - to help others own and grow their greatness in Heart, Body, and Mind! She is a survivor and trailblazer who knows firsthand the strife of living with diabetes and other health issues. Gail has battled diabetes for over 20 years without the use of traditional medication. She believes she has "reversed" her diabetes diagnosis.

Her mission and ultimate goal is to give her clients and readers the tools to confront and move past their fears, overcome obstacles, inspire healthy habits and progressively move toward a healthy lifestyle! Her satisfaction only comes when each client and reader is finally able to create the mental and physical transformation they have always dreamed of, both personal and professionally. This lifestyle will propel you toward becoming the person you always dreamed you could be.

Gail is the Owner and President of Kaizen Lifestyle, LLC. She received a Bachelor of Science - Psychology from Ohio University, and Masters of Education from Cleveland State University. She is an Herbalist and certified as Nutritional and Advanced Sports Advisor. She has been a Social Worker, Educator, Counselor, and Business Owner for over 25 years.

Gail is married to the love of her life, John. She has a daughter, two stepchildren, and a most precious granddaughter.

Gail is making her mark in society. She calculates every step in her business with utmost care and precision, as she steadfastly moves toward creating a nationwide and, ultimately, global movement - to spread the word of living a healthy and balanced lifestyle by her compelling mantra: Truth, Love, and Gratitude. She lives her life as though she is writing her obituary and boldly calls others to that mindset.

DISCLAIMER

This book is based on the author's personal opinion, research and experience. This text should only be used as a general guide or reference for exploring ideas and not as the ultimate source or substitution for personal health, wellness, supplement, physical activity, medication or otherwise. The information given here is not intended to cure, diagnose, treat or prevent any disease(s) or medical condition(s).

MEDICAL DISCLAIMER: All content found in this book, including text, images, audio, or other formats were created for informational purposes only. The content is not intended to be a substitute for professional medical advice, diagnosis, medication(s), cure, prevention or treatment. Do not self-diagnose. Always seek the advice of your medical physician or other qualified health provider with any questions you may have regarding your medical condition, allergies, current medication(s) or other health-related issues/concerns. If you are currently taking pharmaceuticals, over the counter medications, and/or natural supplements, you must consult with your doctor before discontinuing, using any additional supplements or changing your diet and exercise regimen. If you wish to try a natural approach, discuss with a medical or natural health professional first. Never disregard professional medical advice or delay in seeking it because of something you have read in this book or any materials offered by staff of Kaizen Lifestyle, LLC.

FOOD DISCLAIMER: Kaizen Lifestyle, LLC has provided recipes, food suggestions, and ingredients as recommendations to use based on commonly available ingredients understood to be gluten-free, vegetarian, safe or healthy alternatives. We cannot guarantee the gluten-free or vegetarian nature of the specific brand or ingredients you obtain or your preparation of the final recipe. Please exercise good judgment in selecting gluten-free or any other ingredients. We define "vegetarian" as not including any animal product, fish/seafood or any products derived from them or any other part of an animal to our knowledge. The recipes included in this book and all materials or presentations may include animal by-products such as eggs, honey and substances derived from them. Please review the recipes carefully to determine your personal preference.

INTRODUCTION

*Why you will love Secrets of a Diabetic -
A Natural Approach to Great Health*

Dear Reader,

    I was motivated to begin my journey of healthy living after I was diagnosed with diabetes at the age of 25. Once diagnosed, I was determined to change my destiny, but had no clue of where and how to begin. Diabetes was not going to take my life in the same fashion it had claimed so many of my family members. Without assistance and guidance from healthcare professionals, I was determined to beat this life-altering disease.

    I am not a medical doctor, but I have spent the last 23 years researching and interviewing healthcare professionals who practice Eastern and Western medicine, attending health and nutrition classes, taking certification courses, and learning through personal trial and error. I will share with you my life lessons that have allowed me to not only defy diabetes and other health concerns, but to also live a life of freedom and love. The results you experience can change your perspective on life and food forever. *Secrets of a Diabetic* is more than just a book about eating healthy to lose weight, increasing energy or reversing diabetes. It is about a life changing transformation, which you too can experience. The name of my business, Kaizen Lifestyle, came to me over 12 years ago as people often asked, *"What diet are you on?"* to which I responded, *"It's not a diet, it's a lifestyle."* Kaizen is a Japanese term meaning constant incremental improvement. Today it sounds cliché; however, 12 years ago, most people were not talking about *"lifestyle,"* it was all about "dieting," and which diet worked best.

The changes I made were more than just a one-week cleanse, 21-day challenge, a trendy temporary diet, or the next sensation. The change involved implementing a *holistic* system: discovering methods to de-stress, understanding the mind-body connection, and that breaking unhealthy habits was not just about food. It also involved a mindset change and breaking free from emotional eating. It included improving sleep habits, eating foods as close to nature as possible, discerning and incorporating appropriate physical activity, and using herbs and supplements as needed. A lifestyle change continues to evolve in order to become permanent habits. It requires constant enhancement and nurturing over time. A healthy lifestyle allows your mind, body and spirit to interact with the world around you, while enhancing who you are. I made comprehensive changes to strengthen and transform my quality of life and health. The aesthetic improvements were an added benefit. The changes I made helped me avoid blindness, amputation, daily insulin injections and heart problems. I wanted to overcome fatigue, headaches, cravings, digestive problems, and high/low blood sugar. This process created the difference in how I perceived life and my relationship with food.

I love life. I love to eat. I love traveling, hiking, shopping, walking on the beach, and eating most of what I want, in moderation. Why could I not have it all and be without ailments or physical disabilities. Being and feeling my best is of utmost importance. I believe I have control over my health, and would prefer not to be sick. I do not want diabetes or any other illness limiting my mobility to travel, work, exercise, socialize or play with my grandchild. I do not want to miss the beautiful view from the top of St. Peter's Basilica because I cannot walk the narrow and winding staircase leading to the top due to poor health and physical limitations. I do not want the inconvenience of having to stop and take medications, or be unable to explore new and fascinating places because I am physically and financially limited.

Due to nature, hereditary and environmental factors, great health is not always possible. What is possible is that we may be able to limit diseases from ever occurring and/or combat them quickly when it does occur by implementing the strategies given here. Research has proven these strategies vital to a healthy lifestyle. We can possibly accomplish this by the secrets I discuss in this book.

How I feel day to day is an indication of how I am treating my body; being aware of your body is a simple thing for us to do. If I am feeling sluggish, I reflect upon the past day. Did I get enough sleep, did I eat too many pastries, or did I drink enough water? Our body tells us what it needs and we must become in tune with it and listen for the signs.

This book began at the urging of a business coach and my Small Business Association mentor, who after reviewing a program workbook I was putting together for my workshop, felt I needed to put it into a book format. My mentor said, "You must share this information with the world; it would be selfish not to." She believed my health struggles and what I endured from the healthcare system is still a daily challenge for most people. My mistakes and accomplishments may inspire your journey. My business coach said, "This book is laid out in a very simple format without all the medical jargon, with real life experiences that most can relate to." The intent of this book is to set the foundation for permanent change. My journey has not been easy because I did not have the foundational information I have laid out in this book. Due to the human factor, there are still challenges at times but I usually return to the basics to reset.

It has been my experience that in order to achieve a permanent wellness change, a mindset shift should occur. Would you build a house without having a solid foundation? Customarily, we diet, cleanse, fast, and detox to lose weight but do not understand how we became overweight in the first place, why it happened, why we are sick as a society and how to avoid the pitfalls. This book gives you that foundational aspect to make better decisions in order to make this a long life, permanent change.

I plead with you to let go of your excuses; stop the guilt, pity, bad habits and blaming your past, and find a source of internal motivation. Initially, my motivation was my daughter. At the time she was a pre-teen who depended on me and I wanted to be around to see her grow, be an active parent to her, see her graduate high school, and attend college. Sadly, to be honest, that still was not incentive enough for me to make long-term changes. Along the way, I had experienced setbacks into my old habits, due to excuses, poor self-esteem, lack of self-love and just busy with the day to day. It was not until I made a mindset shift, made it an *internal* motivation, and I made it about me is when the conversion took place. I did not like having acne, balding, fainting, fatigue, or the idea of possibly going blind. It was not until I put the focus on me, that things began to fall into place.

Zig Ziglar says, "It's the measure of your attitude, not your altitude that, will determine your success." I had to change my attitude about what I wanted my life to be and shift my mindset. I could no longer blame my past traumas for the lack of self-love. I had to overcome my mental barriers and become intentional with my actions. As selfish as it may sound, I had to develop a motivation bigger than "my daughter"; I had to do it for me. It is not a matter of being selfish, but implementing self-care. I believe God put my body on loan to me, and in order to live the life He intended for me, I must have the stamina, self-love, self-control and self-discipline to give my body what it needs; therefore, my body is able to give me what I need and to embrace life to the fullest.

Furthermore, we must understand that lifestyle changes and achieving better health are possible, though not an overnight process. We did not end up where we are overnight and we should not expect an immediate solution. I am not some health nut or foodie. I do not consider myself vegan, vegetarian, or any other labels and I do not follow any particular diet fad. Diet implies restrictions and strict dietary rules and guidelines. I prefer not to attach myself to any one label or absolute. I prefer to be able make conscious and informed decisions to eat whatever I desire in moderation and to do what serves my body well. I do so without guilt because I am not holding myself to one particular "diet" style.

Now that my health concerns are manageable, I have the luxury of a flexible lifestyle. I maintain a 95%-5% standard; primarily eating fish, vegetables, legumes, and occasionally other meat products, i.e. lamb or turkey. I eat 2-3 meals and 2-4 small snacks per day, consisting of fruits and nuts. Occasionally I have other snacks such as rice crackers, popcorn, sardines or smoked oysters. I drink approximately 60-70 ounces of water daily, which include 2-3 cups of various herbal teas per day. I limit all processed food, canned and boxed food, ice cream, cookies, pastries, sugar and dairy.

A lifestyle choice entails a long-term commitment to making constant change and improvements. There are improvements I continue to make, as I grow older. As our bodies and systems change with age, we must evolve accordingly. We must resolve in a proactive manner to preserve our mind, body, and spirit. It is acceptable to live in the moment, eating whatever you want in moderation and not at the expense of your future state of mind and health.

In this book, you will gain the secrets to change your life forever using a simple four-step approach; Mental Detox, Food for Life, Build Habits Not Equipment, and Natural Healing through food, herbs and supplements. These secrets came from a diabetic's determination not to die prematurely while attending "the school of hard knocks". I uncovered these strategies through research, trial and error, attending health classes, interviewing healthcare professionals, and putting the pieces of the puzzle together. The book is laid out in the sequence I wish I had approached in reversing my diabetes. I believe it would have expedited the process and made my lifestyle change easier if I had gone about it as outlined here. At the time, I did not know what I did not know. When I started, I did not have nutrition coaches or as much research data at my disposal as

I do today. You cannot change what you do not know, but once you become aware, it is up to you to make the appropriate changes.

My prayer is that this book serves you well; use it as a resource guide with the pages dog-eared and highlighted. I am giving you the information all in one place, in a very simplistic format. Therefore, you can begin to make the changes regardless of where you are in your holistic lifestyle journey. You can start the process as you're going through the book, step-by-step or you can read it completely before starting, it's all your decision. It is likely for an individual to begin experiencing positive changes within the first few weeks of starting the process. Wherever you begin, may this book serve your mind, body, health, and spirit.

A Prescription for Better Living

Regardless of where you are in your life's journey, this book can help. The information is laid out in baby steps to set a solid foundation for your wellness journey. It will help you identify how to build better dietary practices by implementing cognitive behavioral techniques which creates purposeful, permanent and intentional healthy habits. The lessons are designed to help you overcome life's challenges, through Mind, Body, Spirit and Natural Healing. You will master how to change those old, bad habits that haunt you, how to stop cravings that can lead to poor eating habits, skin conditions, weight gain, migraines, high blood pressure, heart disease, and diabetes. You will begin to understand food is your best friend not the enemy. You will discover how to choose better foods, love what you eat, understand your cravings and how to satisfy them in a healthy manner. You will have time to do the things beneficial to your health. No more excuses that you did not have the time to cook; I will show you how it is possible even on a busy or limited schedule. You will separate the pros from the cons regarding stress management. You will begin to incorporate purposeful stress management techniques.

Moreover, I am sharing my personal journey and struggles because it is likely they are very similar to yours or a loved one's. You may feel as stuck and alone as I once did, otherwise you would not have chosen to read this book. Please know you are not alone. The path to discovering a renewed way of life does not have to be a solo trip. I am a very private person, but I am choosing transparency because it is my belief that my mission is to help resolve the health struggles we face as a society. I want you to stop hurting and live a life free of illness, pain and suffering. I want you to live the purposeful and healthy life God intended for you. I am not aware of anyone who says, "I like taking various medications," "I like being in pain," "I like sticking myself with needles of insulin," "I like not being able to actively play with my kids," "I like having to do dialysis," or "I like having my limbs amputated." What kind of life do you want and desire?

My goal for you is to love yourself enough to live a long and disease-free life. To free yourself of any feelings of guilt, shame, and self-harm, to be able to walk down the aisle at your son or daughter's wedding or play with your grandchildren. These strategies can help you stop the self-doubt and eliminate your excuses. Most people say publicly, "I love myself," when in reality, if they look closely, their lives and health do not reflect that. I want you to be able to say those words and mean them. Most women are busy taking care of loved their ones. Think of how good you feel when you take care of you. During this journey, you may fall back into negative behaviors. When you become stuck, continue to move forward, keep your eyes on the prize, and keep your goals in front of you, daily. Those unhealthy behaviors may feel good temporarily, but think of the potential negative impact it could have on your wellness. Do not allow those negative thoughts to steal your momentum or aspirations and ensure you do at least one thing each day towards being a better you.

Beware; I will probably step on your toes with some of the things I say here. If that happens, acknowledge it and continue. Most likely, that is where your pain lies and needs the most healing. Therefore, I am asking you to challenge yourself to create change. This information explores how to make changes to suit your lifestyle. When you follow this program as outlined, you begin to nurture yourself from the inside out; physical differences will become apparent, and you will begin to feel healthier within weeks.

This is not a diet book or an easy, quick weight loss plan. If this is what you desire, this is not the book for you. If you are seeking a permanent lifestyle change and health improvement, this is it. This book will teach you how to get started on the path toward building healthy habits that will last a lifetime. I ask that you not form opinions or beat yourself up. This is not the time to get frustrated, but a time to have an open mind, let the past be in the past, and look toward a bright future. Know that it's possible to alter most health outcomes by changing your mindset, behaviors, and habits, if you are willing to travel this road with me.

Below I have outlined the topics discussed in the book. If you are on medications, consult with your healthcare professional before making changes, in order to make adjustments as necessary. DO NOT make medication changes without consulting a medical/healthcare professional.

"Your beliefs become your thoughts; your thoughts become your words. Your words become your actions, your actions become your habits, your habits become your values, and your values become your destiny." - Mahatma Gandhi

Secret One: Be Calm - Your Life Depends On It

Changing your "weighs" to improve your life: As women, universally we put ourselves last, spending time taking care of everyone and everything other than ourselves. We say, "I am putting my life on hold to take care of my children," or "My family comes first." In essence, you are saying to them, you do not have enough self-love to take care of "you." You may not realize it, but this indirect message is contradictory in so many ways to what you probably want to teach your child(ren). Studies show this indirect behavior teaches children how not to embrace self-love on so many levels. Children model what they see. Therefore, if you want to teach your children to have a positive self-image – to truly love and respect themselves - it has to start with how you treat your own body, what you eat, your health and showing self-love and self-respect. In this regard, deciding to change your ways will also help change your "weighs."

It's all about you: Life happens. How can you take back your power? This is not an easy road to travel. Remember, wellness it is not a destination, it is a journey. The bumps you encounter in the road are only speed bumps. It can slow you down but not stop you. This section gives you the blueprint to begin the process by calming your mind, how we perceive problems and events, the importance of forgiveness, and alone time. Certainly, the things I will share with you are those I wish I had known earlier in my life. Now that I have implemented stress management strategies, it has made all other aspect of life much easier. We resist healthy practices and accept stress as a natural part of life. When ensuring proper maintenance of our mind, body and spirit, they are the primary components we need to achieve a most favorable life.

Attending to your inner being, you will be grounded in your space and thoughts, and you will become reconnected with life. This section will focus primarily on three aspects: Alone Time, Meditation and Sleep. These will help improve overall stress management and allow positive energy and good health to easily flow into your life. There is a saying, "You attract what you think and do." You will discover the importance of *me time*, why it is critical and how to make it possible. Do you feel there is not enough time in a day to get things done; you want to have alone time and more sleep? This will soon change and you will design the life you desire.

"Happiness is when what you think, what you say, and what you do are in harmony." - Mahatma Gandhi

We become our thoughts: As a society, I do not believe we put enough emphasis on the benefits of meditation. If so, I do not believe we would have over 264 million prescriptions as, of 2011, written for antidepressants. In this book, we will explore the benefits and the importance of meditation - meditating daily is necessary and attainable in today's busy world. Within these three components, you will uncover the mystery of reducing stress. Stress has earned its name and reputation as a silent killer. Research shows we are productive and motivated in our work and personal life, less sick, and more energized when we manage stress. These three components are strategies that cost you nothing and it's priceless to your health. They have shown to improve your health and in turn, increase your lifespan.

We hold the key in our behaviors, thoughts and perceptions. Our perception allows good or bad stress to control our thoughts and take over our lives. Our mind is the most powerful tool to solve our health concerns. Buddhism is one of several religions that emphasizes meditation and practices mind over body. You can practice meditation without making claims to any particular religion. Studies have tested people using mind over body techniques; they sit on a block of ice and use the brain to create heat within the body to be able to melt the ice. Can you believe the power we have right at our disposal? Once you understand your thought process and how it affects the nervous system, you can unlock the doors to better health.

Sleep does a body good: Adequate sleep has always been a hot topic; some of you may even boast that you function well on very little sleep. This book will explain why a lack of sleep could be the root of all evils. Sleep is something to look forward to enjoying, it is a necessary time for the body to heal, and your mind to recover and rejuvenate from the daily grind. The principles presented in this book are to provide ways to build and strengthen your nervous system. These are the keys to all connected and interacting bodily parts, which allows optimum quality of life. What you do to support it at all levels for life is critical: mentally, physically, emotionally, and spiritually. Regulating stress levels, good nutrition, a strong immune system, and daily physical activity are required for better health.

Secret Two: Food for Life

Cooking 101: The top reasons most people say they do not cook are lack of cooking skills and not enough time. Yet, studies show that Americans spend more time watching the Food Network channel than actually preparing their own meals. Over time, as a society, we have allowed the food industry to fatten us and weaken quality family ties, creating a displacement of home cooked meals and more microwavable options. In 1900, 2% of meals were eaten outside the home. In 2010, 58% of meals were eaten away from home, with one in five breakfasts from McDonald's.

One of the many advantages to cooking your own meal is that you know exactly what is in it. Remember my childhood story: We ate all-natural meats, fruit and vegetables directly from our backyard, and made homemade meals and desserts. Yet, my grandmother still suffered from diabetes. Why was this? Keep in mind that even with homemade foods, we tend to still use processed items like white sugar, deli meat, bacon, iodized salt, white flour, margarine, canned tomatoes, ketchup, milk, lard, fructose and/or corn syrup, artificial color, artificial sweeteners and hydrogenated this and that. Therefore, it is of the utmost importance to pay attention to the ingredients you are using when making "healthier" home-cooked meals, treats, or snacks.

Eating FATS is good: Did you ever think you would hear someone say it is okay to eat fats? In the past, many healthcare professionals have said, "Do not eat fats; it's not good for you." In recent years, this has changed with the realization that our body's make up includes fat cells and we need essential fats for energy. The key is eating good, heart-healthy fats found in foods such as nuts, avocados, olive oil, coconut oil, fish, and seeds, all in moderation.

Secret Three: Eat to Lose - The Power of Food

Eat to be slim: You will find when eating rich foods, you can lose weight and attain radiant health. I discovered a way to eat and indulge in *"treat"* foods without feeling bad, deprived, or restricted – and still be healthy. You will explore strategies not to overeat; it is very important to enjoy your food and be passionate about what you are eating. Studies have shown when you enjoy your food without guilt afterwards, it releases "happy chemicals" i.e. serotonin, endorphins, and dopamine. These "happy chemicals" have a positive effect on motivation, productivity, self-esteem, well-being and metabolism.

Contrary to research, many people still think one of the best ways to lose weight is by starvation, which has harmful health effects. When you stop eating, you are not taking in sufficient daily nutrients; therefore, the body begins to starve and enters a flight or fight state. As a result, the body becomes deprived of vital nutrients and minerals, the metabolism slows down and fat is stored for energy. Keeping the metabolism active to convert food to energy is ideal for optimal body function. This includes eating nutrient-rich foods and foods that stimulate the metabolism, in addition to maintaining an active lifestyle.

Know your calories: It is important to know where your calories come from. However, I do not focus on counting calories - instead, count meals. As a society, many of us have become preoccupied with trivial eating behaviors and counting calories is one of them. I do not know about you, but it is very difficult and tedious to count calories in everything we eat; for me, trying to keep track was nearly impossible and frustrating. Instead, you will discover how to eat nutrient-rich foods and practice portion control. What you eat or do not eat will inevitably have an effect on your health, good or bad. In addition, when we allow ourselves to become hungry, in many instances this is when we overeat or grab quick and easy processed foods that could be harmful to our health. I do not have to tell you what happens when you eat fast foods, processed foods and unbalanced meals.

Secret Four: Get Movin' - Build Habits Not Equipment

Lose weight without ever going to a gym: Diet and exercise are both crucial to a long term healthy lifestyle. In the words of Shawn Talbott, "You can't out exercise a bad diet." Since the beginning, humans have always been active. We were hunters, gatherers and caregivers with active lives. The body was built to move, not sit at a desk all day. We are all different and the body responds differently to various activities. What is consistent is the importance to have some form of physical activity on a daily basis in order to revitalize the body, build strong bones, and rejuvenate the brain. Physical activity has been proven to relieve depression, stress and joint pain among many other concerns.

Exercising does not have to be all-out grueling, strenuous or complicated to be beneficial. We have come to believe that doing an all-out intense and lengthy workout is necessary to achieve weight loss and health benefits. Many experts say we need about 15-30 minute of aerobic (fat burning) exercise that is typically 50%-75%, above your resting heart rate, 3-5 times a week and 1-2 times per week beyond 85% of your heart rate for optimum health. This can be achieved using body weight movement, known as calisthenics; the most beneficial movements are squats, planks, pushups and pull-ups. Typically, any exercise beyond 75% of your resting heart rate on a daily basis could be reversing the health benefits and aging the body faster.

In addition to burning calories, physical activity helps transform the mind. It releases "happy chemicals" and ensures blood circulation. Find the best workout activity and environment for you. It does not necessarily mean a gym membership. Take advantage of the outdoors when possible. Identify activities that you enjoy, indoor or outdoor; walking, running, yoga, Zumba, paddle boarding, raking leaves, throwing a football, hiking, biking, rollerblading, volleyball, or dancing. Get the family involved if possible. Movement is an invaluable part of this process. Make a commitment to being active and just keep moving daily.

Create the body you want to live in: One of the best ways to be active and live the life you desire is to have better health by changing your overall perspective and way of living. The body only functions as well as we treat it. The main goal of exercise should not be to lose weight. Many people get on the treadmill and focus on how many calories they burned. Can you burn off 1,217 calories (the number of calories in an 8 oz. bag of potato chips) in a 45-minute session? The answer is no. Therefore, how many calories burned during exercise becomes a self-defeating behavior for many. When you do this, you believe your hard work is not paying off; yet, your eating habits have not changed.

One single chocolate chip has approximately 78 calories each; multiply that by how many you eat in just one serving. Are you burning that many calories in a 60-minute workout? Studies show that as a rule of thumb, weight loss is generally 75% diet and 25% exercise. Do understand that physical activity is essential to your overall health and weight loss is a by-product of it. Up until a few years ago, it did not take much for a child to get outside and play, but with today's technology, electronics are a distraction and more people are less physically active. In addition, if they see mom and dad living a sedentary lifestyle with a disdain for physical activity, it becomes a part of their belief system. They become less motivated to be physically active and are creating a world of future problems. You cannot change the laws of physics, we get out what we put into our mind and body; junk in is junk out. Do you want to look and feel better? Be mindful of what you are putting in and how you are treating your body. Also, ask yourself what unhealthy behaviors are you modeling for your children?

Secret Five: Natural Healing

"Why not me?" This is not an easy road, it is not a simple, quick fix with a pill, and Lord knows many days I wish there was something I could do to make my ailments go away. I spent many days saying, "Lord why me?" but I have come to accept my ailments and instead say, "Why not me?" If I did not encounter these challenges, I may not be able to hold a space in your life right now. There is a song by Laura Story called "Blessings." It denotes that our blessings come even when we think it is a negative situation. What if my blessings came from overcoming diabetes and being able to touch someone's life? Who am I to say, "Why me?" We cannot change the hands of time, but we can change what we do now and move forward. Many people, although overweight or obese, say "I will wait until I have symptoms," "Nothing is wrong with me," or "I eat whatever I want until I am sick." Yet, they may be experiencing symptoms, such as insomnia, skin problems, digestive issues, weight gain, hormonal imbalance, thyroids, arthritis and fatigue. What you do not acknowledge is that those symptoms can be the precursor to bigger issues to come. Why wait until you have a formal diagnosis; I believe an ounce of prevention is better than a pound of cure. Do not wait until sickness arises before you engage in physical activity, eat nutritious food or use herbs to nourish the body.

Medicinal purposes: There has been a welcome change in recent years; more conventional medicine practitioners are using eastern and holistic approaches. Some conventional healthcare professionals are beginning to acknowledge that patients want natural alternatives. They want to be educated and empowered with natural alternatives instead of only being prescribed synthetic medications. It is my findings that many conventional practitioners are not concerned with preventive care; they are concerned with illness and prescribing synthetic medications, which in many cases do most harm than good. Occasionally, we may need prescription medication but it should be an emergency and short-term. Unfortunately, many people find themselves using these medications on a long-term basis, only to be faced with additional health concerns, due to side effects by the initial medication. Many of us look for an instant cure in synthetic medication; instead, we may be putting ourselves at further harm. Herbs are not intended for emergency use, but taken over time, can reduce emergencies and bring the body back in balance.

People have used herbs for medicinal purposes for thousands of years. However, supplements have only been around the last few decades. The Food and Drug Administration (FDA) does not apply the same level of scientific scrutiny or imposed regulations to supplements as with herbs and prescription pharmaceuticals. Manufacturers of herbs and other supplements must follow good manufacturing practices to ensure consistency and meet quality standards. With that said, it is important for you to perform due diligence in researching the herbs and supplements of your choice. Currently, there are approximately five parent companies making supplements and there are many variations of quality and brands under those companies. Not all supplements are equal - know what you are taking, know the possible side effects and determine if it's a quality product.

The effectiveness of supplements and the impact they have on the body has been debated among nutritionists. I think we have misled ourselves into believing that they are a natural whole food product. Most often, these supplements are items processed in a lab. Iron from a capsule is not the same as iron obtained from red meat or herbs such as yellowdock. Supplements are useful at times but they are not identical to nature's food or herbs. Exercise caution when using some supplements due to their unnatural and synthetic form. It is imperative to seek the guidance of a healthcare professional when using herbs and supplements to bring the body back into balance. I will discuss how herbs, teas and supplements are shown to have many positive effects and natural healing agents. Most herbs are used on a long-term basis while some should only be for short-term use. Some herbs can have negative effects although less likely and less severe than with prescription medication.

Eating right for your lifestyle: Eating better foods helped my organs and body function at its best without the use of medication. Healthy lifestyle practices have helped me to eliminate sinus infections, seasonal allergies, arthritis, colds and the flu. I have encountered less headaches and body aches, reversed diabetes and other health concerns. It matters to me how I take care of the body God has blessed me with. The food you eat should be close to its natural state as possible. "Diet" and overcomplicated eating rules often hinder us. A general rule of thumb is to keep it simple and eat what's right for your body. When we know what we are eating is not natural and making us sick, we should not be eating it or feeding it to our family.

Reprogramming the body: This book is designed to help create an intentional lifestyle and to makeover the body from the inside out. I strive to inspire, motivate and empower you to live without pain, sickness and pharmaceutics. Stop telling yourself "I don't have the willpower"; it's a matter of wanting a healthier life bad enough and changing your mindset. Having a stronger will power does not mean that you will never feel aches and pain, have a health crisis or catch a cold. What it does mean is that sickness can occur less often and when it does, recovery can be faster and you will be prepared with the tools to help yourself.

Reversing the damage already caused will not be an overnight activity. When you provide the human body with the necessary vitamins, minerals, enzymes and other nutrients it needs from the most natural sources, it is perfectly capable of healing itself. Genetically, we are different. We will discover what works best for your individual need and lifestyle. I encourage you to try different options. Do not believe it is necessary to accept a label of vegan, vegetarian or anything else to become healthier. Modifying how you eat does not mean you will never eat cheese, pie, cake, chocolate or white bread. What it does mean is that you will come to a point where the desire and cravings for anything processed will dissipate. If you do indulge, it will be without guilt, in moderation, and not out of habit. It is possible to reprogram the body not to crave unhealthy food; your taste buds can eventually change and the desire to eat unhealthy can diminish. You can achieve results beyond your imagination, which can be transformational. You can gain tremendous benefits from creating positive habits that fit your lifestyle. The goal is to implement all four secrets simultaneously on a daily basis for optimum results. However, even if you start with only one aspect, you can achieve some benefits. Any positive change is better than no change.

I suggest that you apply the secrets in every aspect of your and your family's life and future generations to come. The results can help you to be a better mother, father, husband, wife, friend, son/daughter, and employee/boss. Studies have shown that healthier people are more productive and effective at work and in personal life. They also feel an abundance of energy, loss of weight and feel happier. You create a snowball effect when you are healthier; you are not sick as often, therefore you are not canceling plans with family and friends or calling off work.

Being healthier can reap financial benefits; possibly spending less money on prescription medication and decreased healthcare costs from medical visits and insurance. This all adds up to savings. Instead of thinking, "I do not have the money to buy and make choices beneficial to my health," think of the possible long-term cost in medical bills, medical procedures, prescription medication, as well as possible day-to-day pain and suffering.

There are many benefits to start practicing healthier behaviors. The goal is not to read this book and put it away to never reference it again. The goal is to take this book wherever you go and use it as a resource, share it with friends and family. It is my hope you continue moving forward from this day on and be the best person you aspire to be. Continual growth and higher goals are your new expectations. Begin to think, eat, and crave for constant improvement. Strive to live the best life possible while continuing to make permanent lifestyle changes. Live passionately and preserve deeper meaning in your personal and professional life. You can sustain a mind, body, and spirit transformation that will last a lifetime. When you begin to understand there are many benefits to better health, it can change your perspective on life and food. You become conscious of the possibilities and realize you have more control over your health than you think. When we take a stand against pharmaceuticals, traditional medicine, and manufactures imposing toxins into our food, clothing and furniture, then I will know this book is truly worth not only my time, but also yours.

Your Accountability Partner & Lifestylist,
Gail

CHAPTER 1

A "Trini" Girl

"Ability is what you're capable of doing. Motivation determines what you do. Attitude determines how well you do it." - Lou Holtz

I spent the first 10 years of my life in Trinidad and Tobago, a southeastern Caribbean country, where locals are referred to as "Trini." I grew up in a middle-class family and I am the last of seven children. My parents left us in the care of my maternal grandparents and extended family when I was two years old, while they relocated to New York City to make a "better" life for the family. In retrospect, those first 10 years were probably the most glorious of my life.

Life was simple, yet fun. I found pleasure in doing simple things like playing in the rain, chasing chickens or climbing a tree to pick fresh mangos. We ate off the land and I took it for granted. I did not see it as valuable of an experience as I do today. We were able to go into our backyard and get almost anything we needed to make a full, "healthy" meal. We had chickens, turkeys, fresh eggs, goats, ducks, fresh herbs, and a variety of tropical fruit trees that included guava, mango, cherries, tamarind, coconut, and bananas. We had the luxury of having fresh goat's or cow's whole milk delivered almost daily. If there was something we did not have, there were local markets similar to today's "farmers' markets" only better, and we purchased fresh-caught fish from the local angler. A neighbor may have had something we needed and we bartered or they gave it to us at no cost. Much of what we ate was clean, natural and healthy.

Coming to America

My humdrum life in a southeastern Caribbean country turned chaotic at the age of 10. Over an eight-year period, my parents slowly relocated our family to the "Big Apple." My sister and I were the last of the seven children to travel to America. We moved to a "brownstone" house in a middle-class residential area of Queens. I no longer had a backyard to play in or fruit trees to climb or eat from; instead of open pastures we played on slabs of concrete. The closest park was several blocks away, and my parents did not allow me to leave the block without adult supervision, which meant I did not go often. I did not have recreational centers at school or within the community; therefore, my activities were restricted to the block we lived - riding bikes or roller skating, playing tag or racing with friends and participating in physical education at school. Yet, I usually found alternative ways to enjoy playtime despite not having a back yard. I did not perceive this as physical activity - it was just "playtime" and fun.

The choices of food also changed. We no longer had the land to eat from; we bought all our food from a supermarket. This was unfamiliar territory and I suffered a culture shock. My mother cooked daily, just as my grandmother used to. However, we ate canned beans, frozen vegetables, fruits, meat, and fish purchased from the grocery store. The food was definitely not the same.

An American Girl

In grade school, I was introduced to snacks such as milk chocolate, candy, potato chips, cookies and store-bought ice cream. We received candy treats for answering a question correctly or exhibiting good behavior. Parents also brought cake, cookies and ice cream for the entire class on their children's birthdays, and it seemed mandatory for all students to participate. In fact, some students ridiculed those whose parents did not provide such birthday treats. We celebrated Valentine's Day, St. Patrick's Day, Easter, and Christmas with some kind of "sweet" treat. Sugar-laden, store-bought foods became my new way of eating and since my mother had not forbidden me from eating them, I did as everyone else and indulged. Good reason, right?

As a teenager, I developed a love for soda and candy bars - the ones with the waffle inside and another with the nuts and caramel. My favorite drink as a young child in Trinidad was water, primarily because it was all I knew; I now craved the soda in the red, white, and blue can. I enjoyed these on a daily basis, several times a day until my mid-20s. Prior to my pre-teen years, we ate homemade treats that contained no high fructose corn syrup and no preservatives. In Trinidad, the only time I was allowed to eat anything sweet was after dinner.

The Unknown

In my late teens, I began having what I now know to be diabetic symptoms. I did not think much of it because I was not fully aware of the symptoms or the risks. During my sophomore year in college, I experienced a fainting spell. While at the hospital healthcare professionals discovered a cyst on my ovary, but this was not the cause of my fainting and no explanation was given as to why I suddenly fainted. I did not know or acknowledge the symptoms I experienced (jitters/shaky sudden cold sweats, dry mouth, and fainting) could have a correlation to diabetes. Actually, I never thought diabetes was possible due to my petite size and young age. Most of my family members who had diabetes were either overweight, older, or consumed alcohol regularly. It was not until after giving birth - once the symptoms became regular and obvious - when I took notice. When I discussed it with my healthcare professionals, they said it was nothing serious. They often stated,

"You do not fit the criteria of a diabetic." I was "too thin" and didn't have any other health concerns.

Ms. Independent

As a young child, I remember being with my grandmother in the kitchen, only because I enjoyed being with her and watching her cook. Although I loved to eat, I never had any interest in mastering the culinary arts. I ate so much my family always said, "I don't know where you're putting all that food." After college, I began living what I thought was a "lavish lifestyle" on a social worker's salary at 22 years old, living independently, and eating out a lot more - mostly fast food. Sometimes I ate at my mother's house because I did not know how nor did I have the desire to cook. I was free, single and living the American dream.

Pregnancy and Motherhood

As I became older, I continued to indulge in "sweets" which was very normal within my peer group. Eating a candy bar and soda for lunch was my daily routine. My eating habits began to change during my pregnancy when my physician suggested I cut back on sweets, but did not say I had to eliminate soda. I did cut back - instead of 2-3 cans a day, I only drank one can. The reason offered by my healthcare professional to cut back on the drinking soda was, "The caffeine is not good for the baby." I did not ask why nor did he give any other explanation. I took the advice about the soda, but continued eating all of my other favorite "sweets" because the he did not say anything about them - I did not know what I did not know.

During my pregnancy I gained 60 pounds. I was confronted with extreme swelling, known as mild edema, in my feet and legs during the second trimester; my healthcare professional told me it was normal. The delivery was more complicated than expected, but overall I had a healthy baby. However, at the age of six months they diagnosed her with asthma and at age 17 with Attention Deficit Hyperactivity Disorder (ADHD). Did my love for sugar and soda combined with a lack of information and knowledge prove harmful to my child or was it genetics? Research shows a possible connection between ADHD and high intakes of sugar and caffeine during pregnancy. In an article published in the June 2003 issue of American Journal of Psychiatry, researchers undertook a thorough review of past studies that focused on pregnant women's lifestyle choices and the subsequent number of ADHD diagnoses in their children. They concluded that the regular ingestion of sugar products could have contributed to ADHD. The problems did not stop there; soon after, she was diagnosed with hypoglycemia. This was shocking considering her age, small stature, and relatively healthy lifestyle. However, she is not currently on any medication and she manages her conditions through diet, herbs and exercise.

Living on a Budget

As a young, single mom in graduate school in the early stage of a new career, I began living on a strict budget. In order to live within my means, I could not eat out as much as when I was single; that meant finding the cheapest processed or fast food. It seemed like the smart thing to do at the time, especially when I could get two tacos for $1 at a famous fast-food restaurant. Eating out regularly was neither within my budget nor helpful to my savings. I was always a "saver" and did not like living paycheck to paycheck without anything going to savings. When I started working, I typically put money into a savings account with a goal of one day purchasing a house. However, every month I found myself taking it out as fast as I was putting it in. When I assessed my expenses, I discovered I was averaging over $400 a month eating out. Sadly, this amount did not include the money already budgeted for groceries. This was appalling.

"Chef Boyardee"

Since I had to cut my food expenses, even eating cheap fast food was not beneficial anymore; we were eating more of it in order to feel full. Therefore, I ate more often at my mother's house instead of spending to buy fast food. When we ate at home, it consisted of boxed, canned, and frozen meals. They were simple, cheap, seemed nutritious, and I did not have to spend hours in the kitchen cooking. I often made boxed mac and cheese, canned spaghetti pasta, and boxed tuna casserole, adding broccoli for vegetables thinking that would make it "healthier." We ate so much canned food my siblings gave me the nickname "Chef Boyardee." Things were good because it was simple and easy or so I thought. On days I did not feel like cooking or did not have much to prepare, I continued to go to my mother's, eat, and, load up on leftovers. In addition, I saved money and ate nutritious meals when I ate at her house.

Where Is My Personal Chef?

I did not know - nor did I want to learn - how to prepare a regular meal. I recall my mother often asking me to help her in the kitchen even as a teenager and I refused every time. She suggested watching her cook even if I did not help, saying, "You have to be able to cook for yourself when you get older." I replied, "I don't need to learn how to cook, I have you."

However, my mother did become somewhat of "personal chef" to me when I was older, with the only caveat being that we had to go to her house to get the food and eat whatever she prepared, most of which we enjoyed. In fact, we were eating at my mother's house so much that one day my daughter asked, "Why do we always have to eat at Ma's house. I want to eat at my house." My mother's cooking

was much better than the boxed and canned food and it was free. I thought, "What is wrong with this child?" I knew it was not because she did not want to see her grandmother or was getting tired of going to her house. For Heaven's sake, she was constantly asking her to live with us, but what I later realized was that with these "complaints," my daughter was simply trying to say that she wanted to get home and play outside or just be able to play with her toys in the comfort of her own home. I had to make a change although I did not know how to accommodate her without us going hungry or broke.

Near Death Experience

My world, and life as I knew it, came to an abrupt halt. One day, while driving home from work with my 4-year-old daughter, I suddenly began to feel shaky and nauseous, began to perspire profusely, and even felt disoriented at moments. This was not the first time I had encountered these types of symptoms, but it was the first time it came on that extreme and rapidly. I felt as though I was going to vomit, pass out, or die. My heart was racing, I had difficulty thinking clearly and I did not know what to do. Looking back, I know what I should have probably done, but in that moment, I just wanted to get home. I suspected my blood sugar was low, so I reached for my purse to dig for a candy bar or something sweet to eat as I frequently did, but there was nothing in my purse or the car. I did not want to stop because it was snowing heavily and I did not want to take my daughter out of the car to go into a store. If you have ever lived in an area where it snows, you know the challenge of getting a small child in and out of the car. Suddenly, my driving became erratic, weaving in and out of lanes. At times, I thought I even blacked out for a few seconds. I thought if I make it home, get something to eat, and lay down for a few minutes the symptoms would eventually dissipate.

I recall feeling overwhelmed with an abundance of emotions. I felt frustrated, ashamed, fearful, and anxious to the point that tears began running down my face. I tried hard not to let her see me cry, but even at four years old, it was obvious to my daughter that something was wrong. She asked, "Mommy, what's wrong? Mommy, what's wrong?" I did not have the energy to answer her. She kept asking and eventually began to cry. I got off the highway thinking if I drove on the streets I could easily pull over and call for help if needed. After exiting the freeway, I saw a gas station, and as much as I did not want to stop, something told me I should. I pulled into the gas station to ask for assistance. The next thing I recalled was waking up in an ambulance, my daughter crying as she rode by my side. The paramedics explained that I went into a diabetic shock. It was a blessing that I got off the freeway and pulled into the gas station when I did or I would have blacked out on the freeway. What began as a normal drive home from work ended up being a life-changing experience.

My Doctors Failed Me

The hospital released me later that night and encouraged me to follow up with my family healthcare professional. The next day I went to my doctor, followed by visits with several other doctors in the subsequent months. After some general testing, healthcare professionals said they were not certain what happened, but I seemed to be "okay" now. They refused to do any further testing or blood work because, they said, "You do not fit the criteria for a diabetic." I was told, "Your blood sugar dropped too low, but it is nothing to worry about, probably a one-time incident." Since I appeared "healthy" in every other aspect, it was not a concern to them. Shortly after this incident, I revisited my blood panel report with another healthcare professional; he noted my LDL (bad) cholesterol was elevated. The recommendation given - limit soda, candy, and anything sweet. Yet, he stated, "When you experience these symptoms, eat a piece of candy or drink orange juice." The healthcare professionals did not give recommendations on how to lower my cholesterol level.

Although my instincts told me differently, I wanted to believe that I was "okay" and I followed the doctor's orders. I continued with my life, but paid more attention to my symptoms to determine the cause. I also started inquiring into my family history. I asked my mother questions since her mother and several of her brothers had died from diabetes-related causes. My mom did not know much about the symptoms or treatment, only telling me my grandmother had a lot of pain and numbness in her legs and was told to avoid sweets.

As time went on, I noticed certain things I ate or certain activities I participated in would cause similar symptoms to what I experienced during that life-changing day in the car. When I ate sweet foods, within a couple of hours I felt shaky and my body temperature increased. I developed dry mouth, urinated more often, and at times felt as if I had to urinate, but could not pass any fluid. I also noticed when I did not eat regularly, the shakiness would recur, coupled with blurred vision, headaches, and dizziness.

The situation became frustrating because I was making some changes along the way that my healthcare professionals recommended and still the symptoms did not subside, they just seemed to be getting worse. I became very anal about having candy bars, peppermints or some kind of food item with me at all times, in my purse, in the house, in the car or at my desk. I did not want a re-occurrence of the near-fatal car incident. I began eating every 2-3 hours to avoid becoming hungry or letting my blood sugar levels drop too low. I noticed when I did this the symptoms decreased.

My diabetic symptoms continued to worsen over a five-year period. I decided it was something I had to live with for the rest of my life. At my annual physical examination, year after year, my healthcare professionals seemed to reach the same conclusion, telling me "you are fine." With age and wisdom, I started to do further research and not put my health and trust in one person's hands. I self-diagnosed as hypoglycemic or diabetic, and began to research alternative methods to relieve the symptoms. In the meantime, I was still determined to find a healthcare professional who would give me a formal diagnosis. Without much knowledge at the time, it was just a guessing game. Although I continued to make changes according to what I learned from research, and the symptoms decreased over time, they did not completely go away. I could not find a healthcare professional to do any testing to give a formal diagnosis. They stated that I did not physically fit the criteria for a diabetic despite informing them of extensive family history and symptoms. They stated they did not think my symptoms were serious enough to warrant further investigation or testing.

Never Give Up

"Our greatest weakness lies in giving up. The most certain way to succeed is always to try just one more time." - Thomas Edison

In 1999 I finally I found a healthcare professional that listened to my concerns and sent me to have a glucose tolerance test. I was ecstatic! Someone was finally willing to listen to me. I arrived at the healthcare office at 8 a.m. to begin testing, which involved having blood drawn and drinking a very sweet, orange-flavored liquid that tasted like syrup. This cycle continued every hour for up to four hours. Two hours into the test, they told me, "We don't see any significant changes," and they wanted to discontinue testing. I begged them to continue because I knew the symptoms I had been experiencing, especially with the amount of sugar they were giving me, would soon return. They reluctantly agreed and continued; less than an hour later, they said my blood sugar was elevated, but it was not what they would consider significant or alarming - and they still wanted to send me home. Whatever they were looking for, they did not think that I met the criteria because I did not reach those levels during the allotted timeframe. I could not believe what was happening. Did I go through all of this for nothing? I tried not to start doubting myself and begged them to continue. Although the symptoms had not occurred, I told them I knew what my reaction was usually like and to give it a little longer. They were kind enough to oblige. By the third hour, they reported my sugar level was even more elevated above the normal range, but they were still ambivalent about making a formal diagnosis. I could not believe what I was hearing and again they were ready to discontinue the testing. I asked them to allow me to sit a while longer before leaving. Shortly, thereafter I began feeling slightly lightheaded and my body temperature increased. From experiences, I knew the symptoms would eventually return and I would soon blackout.

The next thing I remembered was lying down on the table in the doctor's office surrounded by my doctor and a nurse, who were giving me fluids through an IV pump, and waving smelling salts at my nose. Soon after, they were giving me orange juice to smell and later crackers to eat. They explained if I smelled the orange juice, it would signal to my brain that food was coming and my blood sugar would start to stabilize. I thought, "Odd, but okay." The doctor thanked me for being in tune with my body. He said without me having that episode in his presence, they would not have been able to diagnose me - scary, but true. Without the episode, I did not fit into the guidelines of what they required for a formal diabetes diagnosis. Today, with those same test results at the two hour mark, I would be considered as pre-diabetic, but back then you were either within the range of diabetic or not.

D - Day

Finally, I received a formal diagnosis - diabetes with hypoglycemic tendency. What was this? In the 90's, discussing hypoglycemia was rare, much less making a connection with diabetes. When given the diagnosis, to my surprise, the healthcare professional simply said, without a blink of an eye, "Okay, watch what you eat, although unlikely it can turn into full diabetes, if you're not careful." After I asked a few more questions and received very vague answers, he later offered me a prescription and I refused. I explained that I had been doing some research and I think I can manage it with my diet, and he responded, "Good luck with that."

Previously, many professionals did not perceive hypoglycemia a serious disease as in recent years. Many healthcare professionals now consider hypoglycemia borderline diabetes. Hypoglycemia is not a medical term I was familiar with, but I was somewhat familiar with diabetes. As a child, my family referred to diabetes as "sugar," but I had no real knowledge of what it meant. I do not recall ever hearing the word hypoglycemia. However, from my research, I understand hypoglycemia as a form of and a potential early onset of diabetes. My observation of diabetes with family members meant being constantly sick, having extreme leg pain, possible numbness and amputation, insulin injection, and ultimately death. I did not suffer any of those symptoms and therefore, I thought I was in a safe zone and could easily control it.

As I moved and changed healthcare professionals over the next few years, I included my new diagnosis in my medical history. Healthcare professionals continued to tell me, "You're too young, too thin, and looked too healthy to have hypoglycemia." They said I probably had some mild case, but not to be concerned. After hearing this often, I took it as good news and I made minimal changes to my lifestyle. My impression was, and most research supported at the time, diabetes occurred mostly in older people, those who were overweight or had very poor eating habits. This was the extent of my knowledge and healthcare providers did not say otherwise. Since I did not fit the diabetic criteria, I thought it would easily resolve over time with some minor changes.

All I had to do was reduce my candy and soda intake, and continue eating regularly, not becoming hungry even if that meant eating an occasional candy bar. Over the next few years, I continued to have irregular symptoms, including constant urination, dry mouth, shakiness, and sweats. It was now the year 2004, and during my annual physical examination with my healthcare provider, he gave me shocking news - based on my blood analysis - I was officially DIABETIC. How could this be? They said I would be fine and did not fit the criteria of a diabetic. The healthcare provider stated I was probably pre-diabetic for many years and it was overlooked. He offered me medication to reduce and maintain my blood sugar levels. Although my future seemed dim and I was very afraid of what could happen, my research showed a history of unpleasant side effects of those medications and I refused them. Research indicated while on mediation patients endured the exact effect of diabetes - other health-related issues, amputated limbs, blindness, and eventually death - as if they did nothing at all. Why would I take something that would not prevent the effects of the disease or resolve it? At that point, I lost my faith in the conventional healthcare system. I was willing to take my chances and continue to find alternative ways to overcome this tragedy. I was newly married and had a daughter that depended on me. There was no way I could allow myself to have any of those problems or die prematurely if I could help it. I wanted to be able to continue living life, as I knew it, without much health concerns, physical limitations or taking prescription medication.

No Respect for Western/Conventional Medicine

After my diagnosis of diabetes, and during one of my earlier encounters, a dietitian said, "Sometimes they make mistakes with those results." She did not believe I could be diabetic and said, "You don't look diabetic." I was so sick of hearing that statement. I thought, "Can someone tell me what does a diabetic look like because thus far they have been wrong about me?" She recommended eating more protein, engaging in regular exercise, taking a multivitamin, and limiting sugar i.e. candy, soda, pastries. I felt as if I was backtracking and reliving what healthcare professionals had been telling me for the past several years. Now even after a formal diagnosis, another healthcare professional did not take my diagnosis seriously nor was able to advise me of anything I was not already doing.

"Goals are achieved with tenacity and perseverance." - Unknown Author

"I Am a Survivor"

After the worthless session with the dietitian, I devoted my free time to finding out more about diabetes. I needed to know everything and anything about it – but more importantly, I needed to figure out how to resolve it without medication. The Internet was now more accessible and I had more information at my fingertips than ever before. I purchased books, spent a lot of time at the library, and took nutrition classes. I purchased my first diabetes related book after I received the hypoglycemia diagnosis, but I did not put much effort into reading it. I put it aside because I did not comprehend the seriousness of hypoglycemia nor did I fully grasp the connection it had with diabetes at the time. When I finally opened the book, it gave me a new perspective on the disease and hope for a better life. If I had read that book years earlier when I purchased it, it may have relieved some of the aggravation and frustration I felt and possibly resolved my symptoms sooner. After reading the book, I realized I had to start making some additional changes to my eating habits and overall way of living if I wanted to extend my life; for me that meant slow, incremental changes (KAIZEN).

It has been a lonely, frustrating, long and at times difficult road to travel. I woke up everyday knowing I had to be conscious of what I was putting into my mouth and how I treated my body if I wanted to control my health concerns and feel energized, instead of feeling lethargic. I became my own advocate, doctor, psychologist, and life and health coach. In addition to my master's degree and experience as a counselor, I earned a certification in nutrition and trained as an herbalist. I learned about herbs, supplements, healthier cooking, exercise, self-love, and stress management in my goal to live symptom-free without medication.

I could not have done this without the help of my husband; at least he made the battle a little easier. He has been my biggest accountability partner, cheerleader, conscience, health adviser and coach. He has been there every step of the way: encouraging me to stay on task when I wanted to give up; inspiring me to cook and be healthier; motivating me to exercise by working out with me; and pushing me to try new variations of activities such as volleyball, softball, belly-dancing classes, and tennis. These were all fun activities I enjoyed without looking at them as exercise. When I was tempted to make bad food choices, he reminded me of the consequences and asked that I consider alternatives. The meaning of my husband's name, John, is "God's gracious gift," and he has fulfilled every aspect of that meaning, especially in supporting me throughout this process.

I am happy to report I have never taken oral medication or insulin. I have periodic low blood sugar, but it is manageable and I know my triggers and how to limit them. I no longer check my sugar levels daily, or monthly for that matter. I no longer experience those traumatic near-death episodes. I am 100% convinced it is due to the lifestyle changes I made over the years, which is what I will share with you. I have learned there is not a "typical' way to look or to feel in order to be afflicted with a disease. People still look at me with doubt and say, "You are the picture of beauty and health. There is no way you are diabetic." What they do not always understand is that I look and feel amazing now because I was determined to change my health status and defy diabetes against all odds. I have been able to reverse this deadly disease and the hold it had over my life; the same is possible for you.

Failure is Not an Option

Many of us do not want to make a change or are afraid we will fail if we try something new. We come to believe we have unchangeable deep-rooted habits. Whether you make an intentional change or not, something will change - for better or for worse. You have to take a risk to change your unwanted habits because the risk of death is perhaps greater if you do not adapt a healthier lifestyle. You must decide what change looks like for you. Someone once told me, "It's in doing, is where you discover." That meant start to do something! You may not have all the answers but in time, it will begin to fall into place and you will discover the answers with every step you take.

This program will empower you with tools and tips to get there. I could not sit around waiting for healthcare professionals to help me; I had to step up and take action because the only help I was given was medication and that was not a viable option for me. I have too many family members who experienced severe complications and some have died even while taking medication for diabetes. I took action by doing the research, reading, and obtaining opinions from holistic healthcare professionals. If I had not taken these steps, I would not have discovered that reversing my health concerns without medication was even possible.

CHAPTER 2

What Is Your Gut Saying?

"Education breeds confidence. Confidence breeds hope. Hope breeds peace."

- Confucius

Most people are devastated when diagnosed with any disease or health concern; diabetes is no exception. Thoughts run rampant through your head. How did this happen? Why me? What caused it and what can I do to get rid of it, fast? The good news is that reversing diabetes, in most cases, is possible if we educate ourselves and take action to change it. According to the National Institute of Diabetes, Digestive, and Kidney Diseases (NIDDK), diabetes affects 25.8 million Americans, while only an estimated 18.8 million are formally diagnosed with type 1 and type 2 diabetes. Unfortunately, the remaining 7 million people are unaware they have diabetes. The Centers for Disease Control and Prevention (CDC) recognizes type 2 diabetes as the 7th leading cause of death in the U.S. and as one of the leading causes of disability.

Diabetes, cancer, heart problems, depression, digestive issues, and hypertension continue to increase at alarming rates. Research shows that every ten seconds someone in the world dies from complications of diabetes. The New England Journal of Medicine suggested that diabetes includes pre-diabetes, hypo- and hyperglycemia, type I, and type 2. Researchers have predicted that there will soon be type 3 diabetes. This category includes autoimmune diseases such as lupus, brain and memory problems, such as Alzheimer's, belly fat and digestive issues. Reversing or managing many of these conditions with little to no medication through your lifestyle choices is possible, with the exception of type 1. Many studies have proven these results, including studies conducted by Cornell University, Cleveland Clinic, and CNN. Although type 1 cannot be cured, in some cases it can be managed with a smaller dosage of medication through lifestyle choices. Achieving great health does not have to be difficult nor does it require medical intervention. The body is designed to heal itself when it's given proper nutrition, adequate sleep and physical activity.

What is Insulin?

Before we get into explaining diabetes and the various types, it is important to clarify and define insulin. Many people think insulin is a liquid substance that is injected into the body - and it is, but these are synthetic forms. Insulin is a hormone, produced naturally in the pancreas that regulates the amount of glucose in the bloodstream. The body uses insulin when glucose rises in the blood stream. Insulin opens the body and brain cells to allow fuel - glucose from the blood stream - for daily life energy. Unlike the body, the brain does not store or manufactures glucose; therefore, it requires a continuous supply of glucose to function on a daily basis. Any excess glucose remaining in the bloodstream after all the other cells receive their supply is stored in the liver and muscles as glycogen.

Insulin plays a major role in the various forms of diabetes. When the pancreas does not produce enough insulin or when the cells cannot appropriately use the glucose that the body produces, it can cause a form of diabetes. As a result, glucose builds up in the bloodstream and does not feed the cells, which causes problems. Leaving any of these conditions untreated over time can result in diabetes and can possibly lead to blindness, kidney disease, nerve disease, heart disease, and stroke. If you are insulin-resistant or have any blood sugar issues, insulin injection or some other form of medication to regulate the sugar levels is usually the primary treatment practiced by most conventional healthcare professionals.

When blood glucose levels rise in the blood stream, it sends a signal to the beta cell in the pancreas to release insulin. Studies show that a lack of or too much insulin production is due to the malfunction of the beta cell. There are several opinions on why this disconnect happens, but the consensus attributes it to a sedentary lifestyle, poor eating habits, and stress. This is exactly the reason step one in this book gives strategies to eliminate or reduce the stress in your life. Research shows that stress can be the precursor for most diseases. It is proven that stress is the number one killer; we discuss this further in Chapter 3.

Now that we understand what insulin is and what it does, let us understand the blood sugar regulatory system and the occurrence of various types of diabetes. The process begins from the food we ingest; glucose is created from all foods. In the Standard American Diet, (SAD) a great portion comes from mostly simple carbohydrates, such as pasties, potatoes, pasta, bread, cookies, potato chips and rice. The digestive system breaks down the food we eat into different sugar molecules, one of which is glucose, and releases them to the blood stream to later become the body's main source of energy. When the blood sugar level rises, it sends a signal and insulin is released. Glucose travels directly into the cells to provide energy; it requires insulin for this process to occur. In other words, a cell would starve from lack of energy if there were no insulin around to signal the release of glucose from the blood stream. In Secret Two, we will discuss which foods you can choose for optimal glucose levels and better health.

What is Your Type?

Now that you have a better understanding of insulin and glucose process, let's talk about the various types of diabetes. This includes hypo- and hyper-glycemia, type 2 and type 1.

Hypoglycemia

Hypoglycemia usually refers to persons with abnormally low levels of blood sugar (glucose) in the bloodstream. Low blood sugar levels signals the pancreas to release another hormone, glucagon. Glucagon signals to the liver to break down the stored glycogen and release glucose back into the bloodstream. Low blood sugar levels can occur due to a malfunction with any of the signals because of other health issues, use of diabetic medication, too much insulin, deficient glucose storage, missed meals, inadequate sugar intake or excessive exercising. Some research suggests that hypoglycemia is not a disease in and of itself, but instead a sign of a health problem commonly linked with diabetes. According to the Diabetic Medicine Journal, they discovered hypoglycemia in patients that are type 2 diabetics and taking diabetes medication. The majority of people know when their blood sugar levels have dropped and have time to do something about it. Whether it is a disease or not, I believe it's grounds to be concerned about your health if it consistently recurs, as was the case with me.

Signs and Symptoms of Hypoglycemia

Many studies state that unmanaged hypoglycemia could be a precursor to diabetes. In most cases, the onset of an episode happens quickly and immediate treatment recommended. Many people look for a quick fix from a candy bar, sports drink, fruit juice, soda or other sugary toxins that may cause further harm. Instead, a piece of fruit, a small piece of peppermint, a drop of peppermint essential oil or a glucose tablet may be a better option, but remember this is not a permanent solution. It is better to eat a balanced meal, when possible, if the occurrence is due to starvation or skipping meals (discussed in Secret Two). Eating will assist the sugar level in the blood stream to rise slowly, back to normal. It is important to speak with a healthcare professional if you experience regular signs of low blood sugar.

According to the American Diabetes Association, typical and early signs of low sugar levels include, but are not exclusive to:

- Trembling
- Shaking
- Nausea
- Pallor (face goes pale)
- Heart palpitations
- Tingling lips
- Sweating or increased body temperature

When hypoglycemia is more severe, the following signs or symptoms are possible:

- Lack of concentration
- Confusion
- Irrational and disorderly behavior (similar to somebody who is drunk)
- Seizures (uncommon)
- Loss of consciousness (uncommon)

Other illnesses or conditions may cause signs and symptoms for hypoglycemia. Healthcare professionals recommend one way to ensure it is hypoglycemia and no other condition is to take a blood test and have a thorough medical evaluation.

What Causes Hypoglycemia?

Various factors from simple over-exhaustion from physical activity to taking too much insulin causes hypoglycemia symptoms. One reason over-exhaustion occurs is due to depletion of glycogen in the muscles and the body cannot maintain the energy for the activity, thus causing hypoglycemia. Hence, the importance of eating healthy, balanced meals is critical when you have a physically active lifestyle. Hypoglycemia could also be a side effect of some diabetic medication. This happens because the liver slows or stops the release of glucose to the blood stream. Another possible cause could be from alcohol abuse, excessive amounts of sugar, caffeine, long-term starvation, missed meals or any other condition that overworks the liver. Overall, hypoglycemia is generally associated with minimal blood glucose, glycogen storage, and possible gastrointestinal (GI) distress.

Hyperglycemia

Unlike hypoglycemia - low blood sugar - hyperglycemia is high blood glucose. Normally, when the blood glucose levels returns to normal, so does the insulin secretion from the pancreas. High blood glucose occurs when the pancreas releases too little insulin or the body is resistant to the effects of insulin, and glucose levels in the bloodstream remain high, resulting in hyperglycemia.

Signs and symptoms of Hyperglycemia may include:

- High blood glucose
- High levels of sugar in the urine
- Frequent urination
- Increased thirst

The symptoms of hyperglycemia sound very similar to type-2 diabetes.

What Causes Hyperglycemia?

Studies show the lack of insulin causes hyperglycemia symptoms. Type 1 and type 2 patients may acquire hyperglycemia if they are not getting enough insulin. Another reason is the body may have enough insulin, but is not using it efficiently due to a breakdown in functioning of the pancreas. Other contributing factors include poor eating habits, lack of exercise, illness, certain medications, hormonal issues and good 'ole stress'. One way to help lower the sugar level is by being mindful of what you are eating and reducing sugar and simple carbohydrate intake. I discuss eating balanced meals and daily sugar allowance in Secret Two.

Hyperglycemia can be a serious problem, resulting in long-term use of medications if left untreated. If you fail to treat hyperglycemia, it can result in a condition known as ketoacidosis, commonly known as a diabetic coma. Ketoacidosis develops when the body does not have enough insulin. Without insulin, your body cannot use glucose for fuel, so it begins breaking down fats to use for energy. When your body breaks down fats and uses it for energy, it is not always a bad thing, normally. When waste products called ketones are produced, the body cannot tolerate large amounts, so it will try to discharge it through the urine. Unfortunately, the body cannot release all the ketones as it does when there is a "normal" insulin level. Therefore, the ketones build up in the blood, which can lead to ketoacidosis. As a precaution, do not exercise if you have ketones. Reports show that exercising when ketones are present may increase the blood glucose level even further. Be sure to talk to a healthcare professional.

Diabetes

Diabetes is a group of metabolic diseases in which a person has high blood glucose, either because insulin production is inadequate or because the body's cells do not respond properly to insulin or both. Diabetes becomes a problem when blood glucose levels increase higher or decrease lower than normal. Sound familiar? It should, as this is similar to hyperglycemia or hypoglycemia. Type 2 is the most common form of diabetes, which makes up 90% of the population diagnosed with diabetes. Recent studies show that many individuals unknowingly experience complications at least 10 years prior to a diabetes diagnosis.

Type 2

If you have type 2 diabetes, referred to as insulin resistance, the body may not be using insulin properly. Initially, the pancreas begins to make extra insulin to make up for the lack of it. Over time with unhealthy habits and continuously high blood sugar levels, the pancreas is not able to keep up and cannot make enough insulin to keep the blood glucose at normal levels.

Some Signs and Symptoms of Type 2:

- Frequent urination
- Excessive thirst
- Increased hunger
- Extreme weight loss or gain
- Exhaustion or weakness
- Lack of interest and concentration
- A tingling sensation or numbness in the hands or feet
- Blurred vision

What Causes Type 2 Diabetes?

The cause of diabetes is largely unknown; many studies identify genetics and lifestyle choices as major determining factors. They link type 2 diabetes to obesity, genetic risk factors and a sedentary lifestyle. Some racial and ethnic groups are also at higher risk. These include American Indians, African Americans, Latinos, Asian Americans, and Pacific Islanders. There is no known way to permanently cure type 2 diabetes, but it can be prevented, controlled or reversed by keeping the level of glucose in the blood within a normal range. The Physician Committee for Responsible Medicine reports that stress management, healthy eating, physical activity and incorporating natural herb and supplements is crucial to the prevention and reversal of diabetes and many other health concerns.

Type 1

Type 1 diabetes, previously known as juvenile diabetes, is usually found in children and young adults. Studies show that approximately 5% of people with diabetes have this form of the disease. In most cases with type 1 diabetics, the body no longer produces insulin because the body's own immune system has attacked and destroyed the pancreatic cells. You may recall from earlier that insulin is a hormone needed to help regulate glucose in the blood stream. I will not delve into type 1 diabetes because there are many variables involved that go beyond the scope of this book. However, many of the signs and symptoms of type 1 are similar to that of type 2; take precaution and get a formal diagnosis from a healthcare professional.

Some Signs and Symptoms of Type 1:

Many of the signs and symptoms typically start at a young age. Most of the symptoms I have found in my research resemble type 2 except:

- Bedwetting in older children who previously did not wet the bed during the night.
- Regular occurrence of a vaginal yeast infection.

What Causes Type 1 Diabetes?

Type 1 diabetes is caused when the pancreatic and beta cells are destroyed and they can no longer produce insulin adequately; this results in insulin dependency, known as diabetes mellitus. In type 1 diabetics, researchers are uncertain what causes the destruction of the pancreatic and beta cells, but it may include genetic risk factors and environmental factors. Several other theories suggest that type 1 diabetes occur when the body's immune system attacks the pancreatic or beta cell. By the time people realize they have a problem, the beta cells have been destroyed beyond repair. Type 1 diabetes typically shows up in children or young adults; because beta cell destruction may take place over several years, it could appear at any age. There is no known way to prevent, permanently cure, or reverse type 1 diabetes. Research shows, when using insulin or other treatment forms to maintain normal blood levels in conjunction with healthier lifestyle choices, as discussed in this book, you can manage the condition to a certain extent. This can result in a reduced dosage of medication and less aggressive pharmaceutical treatments, which can lead to life extension and limited side effects.

The Next Diabetes Epidemic-Type 3

Many experts are calling for a new category of diabetes - type 3, which covers a broad spectrum including Alzheimer's. Researchers at Brown Medical School and Rhode Island Hospital discovered that insulin could possibly be released from the brain and not just the pancreas. This opens a whole new perspective on both diabetes and Alzheimer's, the progressive degenerative disorder that causes loss of memory, intellectual incapacity, and personality changes. Due to the relatively new classification and limited research of type 3 diabetes, I will not go into much detail as this research continues to develop. Following the strategies in this book, using it as a foundation, and building upon them to create a healthier lifestyle can assist with managing issues within type 3 diabetes.

Pre-Diabetes

Pre-diabetes is a relatively new term that has emerged in the last few years. Healthcare professionals refer to it as pre-diabetes because the testing levels are in the early stage of diabetes according to the defined range. Many of my clients and people I have met disclosed that this diagnosis creates confusion and gives them a false sense of the seriousness of the disease. It is like saying pre-pregnant; you are either pregnant or not. Likewise, you are either diabetic or not.

Be certain to talk with a healthcare professional if you realize any signs or symptoms related to diabetes or any health conditions. There are several tests to make a formal diagnosis, find the right one for you: Fasting Plasma Glucose Test, Oral Glucose Tolerance Test and the A1C. If you are not certain about your symptoms, there is a self-assessment offered by the American Diabetes Association you can obtain through a link on their website or my website. Please DO NOT use this as a final or formal diagnosis - always consult a healthcare professional.

The levels between pre-diabetic and diabetic are as follows:

	Pre-Diabetic	**Type 2 Diabetic**
• Fasting glucose	100 - 125 mg/dl	126 mg/dl or higher
• Oral tolerance	140 - 199 mg/dl	200 mg/dl or higher
• A1C	5.7% - 6.4%	6.5% or higher

The contributing factors can be any of the following or a combination thereof:

- Poor diet
- Lack of physical activity
- Overweight
- Constant stress

Listen to your body, recognize changes, and record symptoms when they occur. I had signs and symptoms of hypo- and later hyperglycemia, prior to the diabetes diagnosis, but I was unable to find a healthcare professional to take my concerns seriously. Eventually, I could no longer ignore the information I discovered during my research and began to make changes by trial and error. Research pointed to the fact that many diseases, including diabetes, starts in the gut. Therefore, I believed if I cleaned up my eating habits, changed how I perceived and dealt with food and stress, engaged in regular physical activity and used natural healing agents, I could heal my body. In doing so, I have not taken any medication in over 20 years. I have been able to reverse my condition and now at 48, I feel better than I did at 28.

The Truth Behind The Numbers

Have you noticed the saturation of advertisements for diabetes medication and test supplies in the past few years? Diabetes has become a hot topic, but not many people are seriously attempting to adopt a new lifestyle for prevention and reversal. The increase in numbers we are seeing year after year reflects that. I believe it is because we are scared into believing that diabetes can't be reversed, it's just genetics, or believe that there is nothing we can do.

There are many studies that show most cases of diabetes (except type 1), heart disease, obesity, kidney disease, arthritis, depression, and many other ailments may be prevented and reversed naturally. Yet, based on medical data, over 4.02 billion prescriptions were written in 2011. There has been an increase in diabetes diagnosis by 41% over a five-year period according to the American Diabetes Association. If the number of prescriptions written is increasing yet disease rates such as diabetes, heart, stroke, and cancer rates are also increasing, where is the missing link? If the medications are not repairing, resolving or reversing the problem, why are we not advocating for a natural alternative versus a quick fix with a pill or needle? That is the million-dollar question. Many studies identify two main reasons: the big pharmaceutical influence and laziness of the average person. My intention is not to snub these companies or label people, but to enlighten and encourage you to wake up and take notice of what is going on around us. It's vital to change your lifestyle and mindset to encourage better health.

I applaud you for taking the time to read this book. It is a testament to your aspiration for better health, healthier society, better food options at more reasonable prices and a better life for you, your family and future generations. If you think it's all hype, I encourage you to read the statistics and do the research. Look at the positive effects that occur when a person adopts a healthier lifestyle to include the components shared here. Worldwide, over 387 million people have diabetes, and nearly half of them do not know it. Diagnosed and undiagnosed, diabetes in the United States alone afflicts 29.1 million people, or 9.3% of the population, over the age of 20 years old. Additionally, 8.1 million people are undiagnosed and have reported symptoms - accounting for an alarming 27.8% of people with undiagnosed diabetes. Undeniably, the statistics surrounding diabetes are very astonishing, especially for a disease that can be prevented and reversed naturally, in most cases.

Food for Thought

When some of the conventional healthcare professionals speak about hypoglycemia, hyperglycemia, type 1, and type 2, they speak as if these are all different diseases, when they really are not. They are each in reference to two important things: blood sugar levels and insulin. Managing these two key commonalities with lifestyle changes can, in most case, help prevent diabetes and diabetes symptoms. Studies have shown living a healthier lifestyle can prevent most diseases, since most disease starts in the gut.

I plead with you to do the research, consult with a medical or natural healthcare provider, and look for natural alternatives, where possible, when prescribed medications. I urge you not to give so much control to one healthcare professional. More importantly, do not wait until you have symptoms or experience a crisis before you make better choices. You may feel your back is against the wall when given a diagnosis of a disease. At that point, you may resort to the conventional methods thinking it will correct the problem fast. In some cases, it may but in other cases with long-term use, it may cause other problems and side effects.

In recent years, the pharmaceutical industry has been sanctioned to explain to the public the side effects of pharmaceuticals, hence the lengthy disclaimers in commercials and advertisements. Many diabetic medications and pharmaceutical treatments have side effects including blindness, kidney failure, amputation, high blood pressure, and heart failure. Ironically, some of the side effects are similar side effects of diabetes if left untreated. Maybe if the pharmaceutical companies spent more money on holistic research and development, it is possible that medication would not have such adverse side effects.

Reports in 2012 estimated drug companies spent more than $3 billion a year in marketing to consumers, compared to $24 billion marketing to healthcare professionals. A large portion of marketing dollars is paid directly to physicians or healthcare facilities prescribing those medications. Ask yourself why they are spending more to market to physicians and not to educate the public or produce medications with minimal side effects. The next time a healthcare professional gives you a prescription, ask them if they have taken money, gifts or any compensation from a pharmaceutical company? If so, how did they use it? Pharmaceutical drugs have a place and time of urgent need. As the consumer, educated yourself on the benefits and side effects, then decide what is best for you - pharmaceutical or alternative treatment.

By incorporating the fundamentals discussed in this book and having a genuine conversation with a healthcare practitioner, prevention of most disease is possible. Your life is ultimately in your hands. It is time we start taking some responsibility for our health and advocate for healthcare professionals to advise of natural alternatives and to participate more in holistic care and less in pharmaceutical medication. In some situations, prescription medication may be necessary and in most cases, it should not be a long-term remedy. It is best to find the safest way to handle a health crisis, and then resume any other changes with the advisement of a healthcare professional.

I am a holistic health practitioner, not a medical doctor. I do have firsthand knowledge of personally overcoming diabetes and several other health concerns, and defying them with the principles shared here. Based on my research and experience, this is my understanding of the information. It is my hope that the information will give you further insight into the signs, symptoms, and causes, in order to make the best resolution to address your health concerns. Make certain you consult with a medical or natural healthcare professional regularly for preventive care.

Now that we have covered the basics, let's reveal how you can revive your body naturally.

CHAPTER 3

Secret One: Be Calm - Your Life Depends On It

All About You

"Being in control of your life and having realistic expectations about your day-to-day challenges are the keys to stress management, which is perhaps the most important ingredient to living a happy, healthy and rewarding life."

- Marilu Henner

One aspect of having optimal quality of life is creating a balanced mind-body connection. This mental and physical connection has been an enigma and has no doubt been controversial for centuries. How do physical experiences affect your thoughts? How do mental experiences affect your body? Whatever your belief is about the mind-body connection, you cannot dispute science. Prior to the mid-1800s, masses linked the state of emotions or the mind to most diseases in the body. They sought natural treatments such as meditation, physical activity, and use of plants and herbs. Over the years, the sale of pharmaceuticals has increased exponentially. During this time, the introduction of bacteria, chemicals and toxins into food, clothing, common building materials and household products also increased, while natural treatment approaches began to decline.

Many became convinced that a prescription could prevent and treat diseases faster and better, disregarding the findings of our ancient ancestors. In recent years, the disturbing high statistics in diabetes, heart risk, certain types of cancer, hormonal issues, depression, anxiety and premature deaths motivated the masses to look for alternative solutions and treatments. Scientists rediscovered what holistic practitioners never deviated from - the link between mind-body and natural treatments. They defined the nervous system as the key to the nerves connecting and interacting between parts of the body. Lately, conventional healthcare professionals are beginning to accept the powerful link between emotional, spiritual, mental and behavioral states, the central nervous system, and their connection to stress and health.

The brain, spinal cord and nerves make up the nervous system, which has three basic functions: receive, interpret and respond. Voluntary and involuntary components in the system transmit signals; it regulates certain body processes, such as the rate of our breathing, heart rate and blood pressure without conscious efforts. It allows us full use of our senses, to experience our world with sight, touch, and smell. Dr. Shai Gozani, founder and CEO of NeuroMetrix, a medical device company, says, "Of all the diseases of the nervous system, the most common difficulty that people have is pain, and much of that is nerve-related." Research shows there are 100 million people who live with some form of chronic pain due to an imbalanced nervous system. By the time you feel pain, the mind-body connection has been out of balance long before and it is now signaling for your attention. Pain is the body's way of communicating that something internally is out of balance.

Without the central nervous system, there could be no life. In essence, that makes it the most important system of the body. Clinical trials have indicated mind-body therapies to be helpful in managing arthritis and other chronic pain conditions. There is also evidence that these therapies can help improve psychological functioning and quality of life, and may help to ease symptoms of other diseases. These findings validate the mind is connected with and impacts the central nervous system. When the system is functioning at an optimal level, typically, the body will work to repair itself and find balance.

Be kind to your nervous system, keep it calm, well fed and protect it from overuse so you can have a greater quality of life. I often make the analogy that our bodies function like automobiles. A car needs all functioning parts working in order to run efficiently. It must have clean oil, good spark plugs, filters, properly inflated tires, periodic tune ups and correct fuel grade. Caring for a car requires preventive maintenance for the engine, transmission and electronic motherboard, which is a car's central nervous system. Only when all of the moving parts are working in unison is the car able to operate at its highest performance. Dirty oil eventually creates sludge, which clogs engine parts, causing harsh wear and tear, and the engine will eventually stop working. The body is similar to a car; the central nervous system requires care and maintenance, or it too can accumulate sludge and stop performing. Keep it maintained and healthy and the body will continue to operate as a fine tuned machine. A healthy nervous system is a vital link to living your best life.

When you begin to experience symptoms or are given a diagnosis of an ailment, it is typically the result of improper maintenance. Do not wait until you feel pain or until a healthcare professional tells you something is wrong before taking care of your mind, body and spirit. Ordinarily, subtle symptoms that may go unnoticed, or you think are common, such as restlessness, headaches, migraines, body pain, and constipation, can be detrimental if left untreated. How you choose to take care of yourself does have an impact on your quality of life - good or bad. We cannot change the law of physics: garbage in, garbage out. The reality is what we put into the mind and body is what we get out. We cannot expect the body to perform efficiently and optimally if we are continually stressed, eating poorly, or lacking adequate sleep. You get to decide the vehicle to drive and its level of performance, by determining how you treat your nervous system. Align the central nervous system to feel centered and recharged.

Stress Kills

"Stress can be anything from the lash of a whip to a passionate kiss." - Hans Selye (Canadian Institute of Stress, co-founder, 1979)

At one point or another, we have all heard that stress kills - although many of us do not take the threat seriously. Physicians and therapists have dubbed stress as a silent killer. Studies show that unmanaged stress is one of the leading causes for many of our health and societal problems, even death. It can be blamed for numerous health epidemics such as sleep deprivation, anxiety, depression, weight gain, heart attack, hypertension, belly fat, drug and/or alcohol abuse and many other illnesses. Nearly everyone can relate to experiencing some stress in his or her lives on any given day. When faced with stress, it produces a "fight or flight" response in the body; for example, increased heart rate and blood pressure. If the body remains in this constant elevated state, it can begin to experience rapid negative changes. Bodily systems such as the heart, blood vessels, immune system, lungs, digestive system, sensory organs, and brain can be affected and illnesses begin to manifest. When endangering the nervous system, you begin to struggle with fatigue, depression, lack of motivation, joint pain and swelling, back pain, decreased physical activity, and sleep disturbances. These are signals that the body's system could be out of balance.

When the mind remains out of balance, it can cause psychological and physiological problems - depression, anxiety, schizophrenia, heart attack, arthritis, insomnia, stroke and diabetes. In most recent years, studies have expanded to look at the effects of trauma on the mind and the nervous system. No one knows for sure how it works, but based on research from dissecting the brain, there is a link between the mind, body and overall health. Many scientists are willing to recognize the connection between mind and body and, therefore, are further examining the concept of healing the whole body from the inside out. An article written by Centrec Care - The Wellness Center, says stress management refers to a wide spectrum of techniques and psychotherapies aimed at controlling a person's levels of stress and improving one's everyday ability to function.

Mind-body treatment focuses on modalities that may promote health, through relaxation, nutrient rich foods and plants, hypnosis, visual imagery, meditation, yoga, sleep and several other techniques. It is important to keep our mind calm in order to maintain a balanced nervous system and to maintain a healthy body. Once you discover the benefit of these tools, achieving better health is possible. You can feel centered, strong and empowered through the most stressful events. We may not know all the intricate aspects of how the mind-body works, but we do know there are voluntary and involuntary nerve controls that send signals throughout the body. It is imperative to begin your health journey with a mindset transformation. Once the mind is in order, everything else can fall into place.

It is essential to develop new habits and techniques to deal with stress and life situations. Break the habit of a couch potato, foregoing physical activity, eating unhealthy food, starving your body of nutrient-rich foods and engaging in obsessive social media involvement - these are the enemies and will wreak havoc on the body, mind and overall well-being. When you are emotionally exhausted, you may feel a lack of energy, flop on the sofa and wallow in your sorrows. We do not acknowledge how these long-term behaviors are counterproductive to a healthy mind and can cause further damage, resulting in the use of medication. By implementing sensible health strategies, you can easily move toward a healthier, new persona. It serves as a strong basis for achieving even greater success in business and personal life.

Get Your Mind Right

"If you take care of your body, it will take care of you." - Tony Horton (P90X)

It is my belief that when we learn to handle and identify the source of stress in our lives accordingly, we are already halfway toward winning the battle in achieving better health and balanced lifestyle. I encourage and empower you to make a move toward such change now: To restore your health, improve food choices, manage stress, use herbs and supplements, and make it a daily goal to be physically active. All of these work hand-in-hand in attaining a healthy lifestyle. Have an open mind and look at the process as an adventure - a journey in the travels of life, not a destination. People commonly think they can get the full benefits of doing one without the other. The truth is you cannot gain full benefits of your labor if you do not implement all aspects of the process. You should not expect to have a balanced life in place by next week.

There is a method to having all four secrets working congruently; it requires practice and baby steps, but you will eventually create a snowball effect. In Stephen Covey's *7 Habits of Highly Effective People*, he says, "Your life doesn't just 'happen'. Whether you know it or not, it is carefully designed by you. The choices, after all, are yours. You choose happiness. You choose sadness. You choose decisiveness. You choose ambivalence. You choose success. You choose failure. You choose courage. You choose fear. Just remember that every moment, every situation provides a new choice. And in doing so, it gives you a perfect opportunity to do things differently to produce more positive results."

Perception is Key: Good Stress, Bad Stress

"You can't make yourself feel positive, but you can choose how to act, and if you choose right, it builds your confidence." - Julien Smith

When life happens, how do you deal with it? Naturally, we tend to overlook how perception of the problem can influence our decisions or reactions. Perception helps us determine if we should be worried or not, is it a good or bad situation; it tells us how we view the situation and our world. We write phantom stories in our head and project feelings or opinions onto a situation based on personal events. In most cases, those feelings or opinions create worry and fear. Perception is one approach that influences the central nervous system and drives everything we do. The truth about fear and perception is realizing our response to events.

How we respond to events determines the level of stress the body experiences through external and internal sensors. External stressors include adverse physical stimulus, pain, hot or cold temperatures, stressful psychological environments, poor working conditions, or abusive relationships. Internal stressors can be disease, infection, inflammation, poor blood circulation, irregular hormones, and obsessive worrying about an event that may or may not occur. This affects how we physically react and change the nervous system.

The level of stress the body endures is also determined by how we perceive stress. There are two types of stress, Eustress (good stress) or Distress (bad stress). The terminology Eustress and Distress was coined by pioneering Austrian-Canadian endocrinologist Hans Selye. The term Eustress denotes "good stress" - and yes, there is such a thing as good stress. The word eustress consists of two parts. The prefix *eu-* derives from the Greek word meaning "well or good" attached to the word stress, it literally means good stress. It is believed that famous American psychologist Richard Lazarus was the first to explore Eustress. Dr. Lazarus is known for his work in the study of human behavior, particularly the relationship between cognitive ability to emotions and stress. He believed it's the positive cognitive response to stress that makes it a healthy action - that is, when it gives us a feeling of fulfillment, a sense of accomplishment or any other positive feelings.

Eustress is not defined by a particular circumstance, but rather by how one *perceives* and *reacts* to that stressor. Have you ever noticed at times you function better and do an outstanding job on a last minute project? That is because you have allotted it your energy and focus, and used it appropriately to get the job done. In this instance, you can perceive the project or situation as "good" stress. Your perception of the situation, determines how you perform. However, if such a situation occurs more frequently, causing you to work late and spend less time with family, you may begin to perceive it negatively, thus creating added stress. How you respond to *the stress* of getting that last-minute project completed depends on your current feeling of control, desirability, environment and timing. If perceived appropriately or positively, it could be a more productive event, giving you a great sense of accomplishment and increasing your confidence. Other types of *good stress* include starting a new job/career, getting married, having a baby or buying a house; these are considered wonderful, memorable, feel-good moments in life.

On the other hand, *Distress*, referred to as "bad stress," includes loss of a job, difficult boss, financial issues or an abusive/difficult relationship. Typically, these things threaten our livelihood and are deemed as stressful. Therefore, we react accordingly; our senses go into "fight or flight" response. Though they are usually the less productive responses, we may become anxious, sad, angry, over eat, or starve in order to cope with the stressors. It is critical to our central nervous system to start practicing separation of the good, bad and ugly. Most of us perceive any stress as distressful, causing us to place good and bad stress into one big stressful category, resulting in internal danger.

How we perceive a situation is key. Remember to deal with both types accordingly, without fear and with clear thoughts toward solutions. Typically, how we identify the situation depends on current feelings of control, desirability, environment and timing. If the response to stress is with a sense of meaning, hope and vigor, the result can be life-enhancing wellness. Generally, how we deal with a stressful situation also depends on how much unresolved stress we have been carrying from the past. To achieve greater wellness, consider changing your perception, look at solutions not the problem, set limits, learn to say no and spend some time alone on a regular basis. It is important to take time and de-stress every day from the daily grind.

Forgiveness or Unforgiveness

"You only have control over three things in your life: the thoughts you think, the images you visualize and the actions you take." - Jack Canfield

Experiences influence our perception of our life and how we treat ourselves. We often carry traumatic events from childhood into adulthood and continue to relive them to the point that they shape our behaviors negatively. Our negative perceptions bring fear, fear brings worry, and worry brings stress; hence, the acronym for FEAR, False Evidence Appearing Real. The repetition of fearful thoughts and situations become our reality. This in turn can result in emotional eating. With that in mind, we have to be willing to forgive those who have hurt us - not for their sake, but for our own. The truth is forgiveness and letting go of guilt, shame and resentment will allow you to heal your mind and achieve better health. Most of all, we must release the negative events from our past and stop using them as excuses to not move forward with better wellness.

I once heard a pastor give a sermon about forgiveness and I loved the simplicity of it. He said there are three misunderstandings about forgiveness:

"Unforgiveness will set you on fire." - Matthew 6:12

- Misunderstanding #1: If I am willing to forgive, it minimizes what happened to me. No, it does not. This allows you to acknowledge what happened and move forward.

- Misunderstanding #2: In order to forgive, I must reconcile with the person. Forgiveness does not mean going back to that person or place. It is just a matter of knowing it within yourself. What if that person has passed away? Does that mean you never forgive? The person does not need to be present nor do the words need to be spoken to them. You just have to know in your heart that you forgave him/her.

- Misunderstanding #3: Forgiveness is about the other person. No, it is not; it is about you. It is not about letting the other person off the hook or letting yourself off the hook, but recognizing that you are past that situation and have moved forward.

A close friend of mine once told me, "Forgiveness is not a feeling. It's a choice." You choose to abolish your past and not allow it to affect your current life. Take time to resolve past traumatic issues, regardless if you were the victim or offender, do not put other things over your mental and physical well-being on a regular basis - forgiveness is a part of your well-being process and decreasing stress factors in your life. I encourage to you make it a weekly exercise during meditation to forgive those who have wronged you and/or who you wronged, past and present.

Childhood-Adulthood: It Takes a Village

"I believe that the greatest gift you can give your family and the world is a healthy you." - Joyce Meyer

At the age of 24, I endured an emotionally abusive relationship, coupled with single-handedly parenting a two-year-old, managing a full-time career as a social worker, buying a house and attending graduate school. Time and time again, I felt suffocated when faced with life matters and it seemed that my world was closing in on me. I hate to admit it, but sometimes I felt like dying and just giving up. Knowing I had to live for my daughter was the only thing that kept me going at times. I felt as if I was running from one thing to the other, and could not catch a break. Immaturity, past traumas and unhealthy relationships clouded my perception, and it caused internal damage.

Most people would agree that such a situation constitutes stress factors. I believe my perception and lack of resources, support system, and knowledge to manage these factors played a part in my poor eating habits. This affected my digestive issues, lack of physical activity, and inadequate sleep, which in turn led to the diagnosis of hypoglycemia and, ultimately, diabetes. Nonetheless, I faced a tremendous amount of stress, good or bad, but I perceived it all as urgent stress. At the onset of symptoms, my body was telling me to slow down and make changes. Unbeknownst to me, my body had been in distress and I was clueless on how to resolve it. This was not something that I learned neither as a child nor as a psychology major. Most families do not talk about stress management and how it relates to health and well-being and my family wasn't any different.

Stressful events affect us throughout life, starting in childhood. The adults in our lives do not give instructions nor do we generally observe modeled behaviors of how to manage stress appropriately. Therefore, we go into adulthood with a lack of knowledge of how to deal with stressful life issues. This creates chaos on our system unless we bring it into balance. Children are normally described as "carefree" because they do not have responsibilities such as bills, relationships, and work. Most adults believe children do not have stress factors unless it is a traumatic event; death of a loved one or divorce, and that could not be further from the truth. The Kids Health Organization describes stress as a function of the demands placed on a person and their ability to meet them. This means that children feel stress when they have a recital, sports competition, school testing, peer pressure, bullying and social isolation. It becomes an untouched subject and we take these unhealthy behaviors and perceptions into adulthood. Oftentimes, adults tell us "life happens" so deal with it. Most children and adults have no knowledge of how to handle or perceive stress or trauma in order to deal with it appropriately, causing our body great harm even from a young age.

As adults, we give in to the pressures that society imposes on us and we try to live up to everyone else's expectations. We get lost in the stressful world of family, bills, work, and other responsibility. As we get older and gain foresight, we still have not learned how to manage or compartmentalize stress, and we tend to bring about unnecessary worry and fear into the equation. Consequently, this changes our perception, creating more fear by projecting negative thoughts and feelings into a situation.

I'm Not Your Superwoman

On the outside, it seemed as if my life was almost perfect. I thought I was managing my life by giving everyone else the best of me and doing it all. Throughout my early twenties, I worked overtime and on weekends to keep up with paperwork and make extra money. I stayed up usually until 2 a.m. completing reports for work or schoolwork, only to awake at 6 a.m. for work. My busy days included volunteering at my daughter's school, food shelters and several other community events. I spent time interacting with my daughter transporting her to various extra-curricular activities while ensuring she socialized with her peers. I spent many days cooking, cleaning, working, studying, and attending church, with little time to myself. My obligations and inability to say no to others became even worse as I became older. I felt I had to be involved and do as much as possible to be a productive citizen. I thought things were under control and I was being a "responsible adult," and that multi-tasking came with the territory called "adulthood."

As mothers, wives, caretakers, and professionals, women are often viewed as androids with boundless energy and, accordingly, we think it is beneficial if we stay busy and learn to multitask. Studies show most people are more unproductive when they multitask. This occurs because you are not focusing on one task as intended;

therefore, it will take longer to get a job done due to distractions. However, if this is all we know and do, we never really allow ourselves to stop, think and alter the behavior. We do not realize even when we attempt to pamper ourselves or have alone time how much we still multitask. For instance, when we get a pedicure, we may be preoccupied with talking on the phone, or taking the children with us. It is important to make time for you - alone, and allow yourself time to de-stress. Women have allowed society to brainwash them into thinking in order to feel or be productive, multitasking and busyness are necessary. We have learned to do and be everything to everyone except ourselves. If you are not caring for yourself, you eventually may not be healthy enough to care for anyone else.

"Strike 'Obligation', Insert: 'Choice'." - Danielle LaPorte

Later, as I improved my ability to juggle life, I decided I could no longer be "superwoman" and became comfortable with saying "no" to taking on so much and started taking care of me. When I changed my opinion of being superwoman, I began to feel a shift in my body. My mood and sleeping patterns improved. Although I was working on the stresses in my life, my body started to react to the mental damage started years prior. I began to experience digestive issues such as constipation, ulcers, and acid reflux.

By and large, we think we have things under control because we have come to accept the craziness and chaos that comes with life. It does not mean the body has immediately turned off the "fight or flight" switch. When I began to have digestive issues, conventional healthcare providers did not suggest behavioral modification methods like meditation, alone time or developing healthy relationships. The only treatment offered was various medications for depression, sleep, anxiety and acid reflux. No one told me these symptoms could be stress related. They did not advise the importance of de-stressing using physical activity, meditation or sleep as treatment options. It was not until I researched how to manage my health issues that I realized my perception of life's problems and the unhealthy coping mechanisms I used were endangering me, my family and other relationships.

You are probably saying to yourself, this sounds good, but you do not know my life. It is true; everyone does have different life situations and unique circumstances. No matter our differences, we all can benefit from acknowledging our situation, deciphering good from bad stress, dealing with them accordingly, and incorporating healthy methods to de-stress daily.

Let Go and Let God

"Accept the things I cannot change; have the courage to change the things that I can; and the wisdom to know the difference." - The Serenity Prayer

Studies show that most people who work long hours and stay continuously preoccupied are actually motivated by a fear of failure. They avoid facing themselves and other aspects of their life they do not want to deal with. Those behaviors ultimately may be the cause of health issues and other unhealthy behaviors. I made a decision to change my perspective and begin to take care of me. I had to recognize the benefits that such a shift would have not just on my emotional, spiritual and physical well-being, but on my family. We have to say "no" sometimes to working late, taking on extra projects, and responsibilities because we are asked. It is time to start saying, "yes" to your sanity and health and, to making better choices to honor you.

You must find time to spend alone and bring balance to your life. Spending 20 minutes for yourself is not going to cause things to fall apart, but will help things fall into place. A positive shift began when I acknowledged the correlation between the creation of life and silencing of the mind, and the positive impact on one's health. Think of how life starts; it is in silence, sitting dormant. A woman carries a baby for months in a protected capsule, like a seed that's planted in soil and remains dormant and undisturbed until it begins to sprout and flourish. We have to treat our minds with this same concept.

We have to let it be silent and recharge before it can effectively think, analyze and process our thoughts. We know health is all about maintaining a healthy mindset. Why are we not practicing it? That is the million-dollar question.

When I understood the importance of keeping the mind still, it became a valuable strategy. I began to incorporate the strategies of cleansing my mind, changing my perception about life and making some alone time. I made a decision that my health and life were too important and immediately put these strategies into practice. I would rather take preventive measures to improve my quality of life and slow down the inevitable.

Me Time

"The more you like yourself, the less you are like anyone else, which makes you unique." - Walt Disney

Make it a daily or weekly habit to do something good for you. Start with baby steps; pick one thing you can do weekly and build upon it as you continue to grow and learn. During this time, choose your thoughts carefully; be mindful of the words you speak and your perception of life. Make certain they are positive and set your intention to a healthy start. Here are a few tips:

- Create a home spa in your bathroom, with scented candles, music, wine and lavender essential oil. Ask your spouse, parents, or best friend to watch the kids for an hour. If not put them to bed early as you relax, enjoy, and take some time to regroup.

- Get a professional massage once per month, if possible. This allows you to distress and release toxins from the body. If you are on a tight budget and cannot afford once a month, save for it and make it a treat a few times a year. If you have a significant other, friend or spouse, ask them to give you a 10-minute massage.

- Set up a spa day at home. Give yourself a facial, nail or foot treatment, wash and style your hair.

- Spend time with a girlfriend, talk to a health/life coach or counselor. Conversation is great with a person you can laugh with and confide in. Talk with someone who will not judge you, but lift you up with encouragement and support.

- Take care of yourself. Feel and look your best. When you look your best, you feel your best. Wear clothes that make you feel good and sexy. You define what sexy means to you. These things help to make you feel better, look better and enhance your confidence.

- Keep a journal. Acknowledge stressful events or situations, move forward and look for solutions. Beware of stressful patterns or events i.e. working late, overloaded schedules, and negative thoughts.

- Take control of your environment. It is okay to say no.

- Sweat it out. Exercise is a great stress reliever and it stimulates happy chemicals in the brain (We will talk about this more in Secret Three). When you cannot do a full workout, take a short walk or run; it releases endorphins, which reduces stress.

- Watch a comedy or read the funnies - laughter is good for the soul and is shown to reduce wrinkles. When was the last time you really had a good, hard laugh?

- Do something that makes you happy like gardening or completing a crossword puzzle.

- Practice deep breathing exercises - helps the body relax, sends oxygen to your cells and calms the central nervous system. Sitting still with your tongue pressed to the roof of your mouth throughout the process; begin to inhale through the nose, with the mouth closed for a slow count of seven. Hold the breath for 2-3 seconds and exhale through the mouth for a slow count of eight. Mindfully repeat this 5-7 times.

- Do gardening or buy a plant - studies found that people with plants experienced an average of a 4-point blood pressure drop.

- Spray your mouth with peppermint; peppermint increases stress-fighting hormones and energizes you.

- Take up a hobby or create an interest group. Remember: Do not sweat the small stuff.

SHOCKING FACT: When stress is managed, research shows we are more productive and motivated. This may sound *insane,* but it's true. It can create confidence, positive self-esteem and productive competition when handled appropriately. We feel good overall and reward ourselves accordingly when stress is conquered. It is no coincidence that "stressed" spelled backward is "desserts" (healthy desserts). Frequently, we cannot turn off the constant stress - but we can shut down the worry, and how we perceive and respond to a situation. Distinguish good stress from bad stress. Find the root of worrying and shut it down by acknowledging it and determine if it is your current reality (situation). If not, dismiss it.

When managing stress and using it appropriately, we can become more efficient and productive in our daily lives; this leads to overall better health and a healthier lifestyle. The key to managing stress is your perception, positive thoughts, behaviors, and sense of self-importance.

CHAPTER 4

Meditation

"The only thing we have control over is our thoughts." - Napoleon Hill

In Western society, I do not believe we place enough emphasis on the benefits of practicing relaxation or meditation. If we did, I do not believe we would have the high number of antidepressant prescriptions, or stress-related deaths as the number one cause of death. Eastern countries practiced meditation for centuries, making its way to the West in recent years. Meditation is more popular and widely accepted today as a healing practice for inner peace, deep relaxation and to strengthen the nervous system. Previously, many people associated meditation with some form of religious belief or cult act. Dr. William C. Bushell, an MIT-affiliated researcher in medical anthropology and director of East-West Research for Tibet House in New York says, "Meditation is a cognitive-behavioral practice that East-West science suggests may be more effective than any existing Western medical intervention."

In Hinduism, they do not consider the act of meditation to be powerful on its own, it is combined with the belief that the central nervous system, small yet powerful beyond measure, is the soul. Recall from the previous chapter, scientists say "There is no life without the central nervous system." Hinduism professes that meditation helps to restore the central nervous system. Meditation helps to move beyond the mind, to release the constant flow of thoughts, emotions, and worries, in order to bring stillness and silence to quiet the mind. It takes you from a state of constriction to peacefulness and light-heartedness, to unlock your greatest potential and creativity.

The central nervous system is paramount to optimum health. Tibetan Lama Phakyab Rinpoche demonstrated that through his act of positive meditation, he maintained thoughts of removing obstacles and gaining protection to heal himself of gangrene. Rinpoche immigrated to the United States in 2003, as a 37-year-old refugee. According an article written in the Daily Beast, his diagnoses were diabetes and Pott's disease. His health was depleting at a rapid rate so much that his right foot and leg developed gangrene. During his hospitalization and subsequent examination by three different doctors in New York City, he received the same treatment recommendation - amputate. There is no known cure for gangrene other than amputation. He expressed that he was more afraid of losing a leg than death. He wanted to try to save his leg if possible. Through the help of the Dalai Lama, he meditated for months. The result: After 10 months, his leg healed and he was walking again. Today a group of doctors at New York University are studying his brain and his act of meditation to make sense of this miracle. This is one of several studies reporting that healing the body through meditation is possible; this healing includes general and physical health. If that does not convince you, studies also reported meditation could make a person look five to twelve years younger.

Every day, we face stress factors, make many decisions and produce many thoughts. We are in the midst of a fast-paced society; setting goals, planning dinner, making career decisions, raising children, managing relationships, dealing with health challenges, job responsibilities - with any and everything that we do, there is a thought behind it, whether positive or negative. Accordingly, we must train our minds to think positively in order to perceive life events as more than just traumatic, unpleasant, unwanted, stressful, busy or chaotic. We must master how to compartmentalize good and bad stress and release it for the benefit of better health. Living in such a rat race, we may wonder if there is such a thing as quiet time. There is, do not lose hope. Take comfort in the word, Matthew 11:28-29: "Come to Me, all you who labor and are heavy-laden and overburdened, and I will cause you to rest. I will ease, relieve and refresh your souls. Take My yoke upon you and learn of Me, for I am gentle and humble in heart, and you will find rest for your souls."

Studies show that meditation and prayer are two superior methods used to accomplish many physical and mental advantages. Your mind will begin to reform and things will begin to change around you, for the better. You will notice subtle changes in the words you choose to use, how you feel, your thoughts and how you respond to life events. This will greatly affect your physical appearance as you begin to change how you treat your body and the food choices you make. Your overall perception of life will begin to transform from the inside out. Meditation is one form of stress management. It does not mean that it protects you from life events; it means you are better prepared to handle them when they arise. When we manage stress, we begin to take charge of our lives, and take back our power. You can reclaim your thoughts, emotions, decisions and the way you work through problems. You will begin to take a stand for a better livelihood. With practice, patience, and persistence, you can learn how to accomplish positive thoughts and meditation even while driving.

Breathe Deep

Usually, we become conscious of our breathing during meditation. Deep breathing allows us to inhale oxygen and exhale the bad toxins. Oxygen nourishes the brain and body cells, and supports the nervous system. It helps reset and reboot our minds, which helps to create a better functioning body. Oxygen increase is one of many benefits to meditation. It helps reduce your stress levels, slow the aging process, increase quality of sleep, improve cognitive functioning and create a greater appreciation for life. The physiological change is stimulated as every cell in the body is oxygenated and given energy. Happy chemicals such as Dopamine, Serotonin, Oxytocin, and Endorphins begin to release. This results in joy, happiness, peace, and enthusiasm. On a mental level, regular meditation calms the brain and brings it to a relaxed state. When the brain relaxes, the nervous system is relaxed and that promotes healing. As the mind restores itself, you can begin to think more clearly. Meditation becomes the birthplace to gain insight, creativity and inspiration.

Physical Benefits of Meditation

On a physical level, benefits include:

- Lower blood pressure
- Lower levels of blood lactate, reducing anxiety attacks
- Decrease tension-related pain, such as tension headaches, ulcers, insomnia, muscle and joint problems
- Stronger immune system
- Increased energy level, improved metabolism, and lose weight

Mental Benefits of Meditation

On a mental level, benefits include:

- Less anxiety
- Better moods
- Reduced stress levels
- Increased attention span
- Emotional stability
- Creativity
- Improved intuition
- Better clarity and peace of mind
- Sharpened mind through increased focus and relaxation
- Reduced tension, anger and frustration

To get the full benefits of meditation, it takes only a few minutes a day, on a regular basis. Meditation can bring clarity, it can cleanse and nourish the soul, and it can bring you true transformation.

Empty the Trash Can

As kids, we played with dolls, taking care of them or other siblings. For many women, we typically grow up to be the caretakers and nurturers for those around us. We learn to take care of others, but all too often, we do not learn to take care of ourselves. We must practice taking care of our "soul" by nurturing it - spending time in prayer, meditating daily and cleaning out the clutter we carry around in our minds and soul. As with a trash can, if you do not empty it when it's full, it spills over and begins to rot. Similarly, the same type of corrosion can happen to the mind and soul if we do not regularly maintain them. This can result in diseases and adverse health conditions in the body.

Many of us have come to accept the fact that life spins out of control and there is very little we can do about it. I am here to tell you yes you can take control. The Bible speaks to this notion in Romans 12:2, *"Do not conform to this world, but be transformed by the renewing of your mind."* You must build a strong "locus of control," and acknowledge that you do have influence over your life. I have found that the best solutions and decisions come to me during meditation. The soul cleanses when thoughts are pure and positive. We cannot control the world around us, but we can control how we react to, perceive it and its effect on us. Perhaps meditation is a far-fetched concept for you, but I still challenge you to try it for a week.

"When you connect to the silence within you, that is when you can make sense of the disturbance going on around you." - Stephen Richards

When I started making changes to my eating habits, it was very difficult. I focused on changing the behaviors, but did not have my mind in alignment with my lifestyle goals. I understood what eating healthy entailed and I realized the challenges that came with it. It appeared to be common sense, but implementing it consistently was a challenge because of all the distractions (busy schedules, work, and family) around me and I allowed circumstance and situations to influence the unwanted behaviors. There was work stress, working late, extended family issues, not having enough time in the day, not having time to cook regularly, financial stress, new marriage, and raising a pre-teen, two new stepchildren, baby mama drama and lots more. I did not have the mental tools to work through my stress factors, as I was being pulled in many directions. I blamed my stress on others and did not accept responsibility for what I was doing to cause it.

I knew I had to make changes to my eating habits to improve my health, but often, I inadvertently slipped back into old habits of fast foods because it was easy; comfort foods tasted good and made me feel better emotionally, or so I thought. It was not until I discovered meditation years later that I realized I allowed stress and emotional baggage to dictate my decisions. I was not taking responsibility for my negative behaviors, it contributed to setbacks, and that made it difficult to make permanent healthy changes. The "busyness" kept me from staying on track and building good habits - I allowed stressful situations to control me and I took my eyes off the primary goal. These things were war against my soul, creating ailments. 1 Peter 2:11 says, "Abstain from sinful desires, which wage war against your soul."

Life Happens

I was preoccupied with the busyness of life, saying yes to everyone else but myself. Nothing was falling into place because when I experienced stress, hurt, disappointment and anger, I resorted to eating fast food and preparing processed food. When emotionally stressed, I sat on the couch watching TV and eating comfort foods such as ice cream, whipped cream, anything chocolate, cookies, candy and sharp cheddar cheese and crackers; although I was lactose intolerant, I did not care how it was affecting my body. I took a pill to ease the bloating and gas, and thought that's all that mattered.

Life happens on some level daily, and we all deal with it differently. Many of you can relate to how I dealt with life events, but it's not the best solution. In my case, it was "bad" food, for others it may be gambling, shopping, drugs or alcohol. When life happens and we feel out of control, most of us resort to unhealthy habits because we have not prepared our minds to deal with it differently. When I discovered meditation, it allowed me to prepare for those times and avoid slipping into old behaviors and thought patterns. The new habits replace the old; once you are better prepared and make a conscious decision of how to cope with life. You do not allow life or other people's behavior to dictate your lifestyle.

We allow life matters to control our mind, body, and spirit and we accept it as part of life. We control many of the things that occur in our lives, yet we do not see it as so. Instead, we say, "I wish I had control" or "I wish I had the willpower to change it." You do have control and the will power; you just haven't tapped into it or wanted whatever that *object* is bad enough. We commonly become content with easing through life, not living intentionally. I believe the Universe contains magnetic energy - what you give out is what you get back, physically, mentally and spiritually. Some may refer to it as Karma; it's one in the same. Karma means action, work or deed. It also refers to the spiritual principle of cause and effect, where intent and actions of an individual (cause) influences the future of that individual (effect), according to Webster Dictionary. Are you being intentional about improving your health?

As a society, we tend to take on too many responsibilities and don't respect our limits - it's okay to say no. We think that being busy all the time is a positive quality, and we glorify being busy, when it negatively affects the nervous system and, ultimately, our health. It is important to identify the source of the stress, be intentional and find solutions instead of repeating the problems, allowing them to persist or choosing to ignore them. Being busy and doing meaningful things is permissible, but when we consistently have chaos in our lives, are busy and unproductive, we allow that to become an excuse for not eating healthy, working out, meditating or spending time alone. It becomes problematic; you feel things are out of control when you are not being intentional about taking care of you or the situation.

I had to carefully manage my stressors and put things into perspective. In doing so, I realized that I needed to slow down and take time for me, and explore ways to calm my mind. It seems like such a simple task, yet it can be difficult for many of us to create the time to spend alone, be alone with our thoughts, and sit in silence. When I started meditating, things started to happen that I could not explain. Money started to flow, financial woes dissipated, John noticed I was calmer, and my health issues began to resolve. People came into my life unexpectedly to assist with my goals such as when an herbalist befriended me and assisted with my health and nutrition at no cost. These were all things I stressed over, but through meditation and prayer, and changing my behaviors, the Universe began to resolve those concerns. Once you get into the practice of meditation and realize the positive effects it can have on your life and those around you, it becomes one of the most powerful tools you possess.

How to Make the Perfect Pound Cake

As part of the American culture, we live for that annual one-week vacation to get caught up on relaxation and quiet time, when most time the vacation is as fast paced and busy as our everyday life. Finding quiet time every day serves you best. Studies show that stress not only affects how we react or feel, but it also changes our hormones, which can wreak havoc on the whole system, recreating the cycle of stress, bad habits, and health issues. I implore you not to wait until you receive an unfavorable diagnosis to make a change in your daily routines.

Rather than take proactive or preventive measures, most of us live in a constant reactive state. Apply positive energy to preventive measures, not always putting out fires. We live in a society that relishes instant gratification and drama, which is one reason why drama and reality shows are so popular. We attempt to lose ourselves in someone else's chaos, hoping not to think of our own. We allow these negative influences - other people's drama - into our mind, which affects how we react and unconsciously cloud our personal decisions. What we do not acknowledge is when we do not attend to our own "drama or chaos" it causes more harm than good, physically and mentally. When we do enter a danger zone, we want an instant result usually with a pill, not realizing those results may come at a larger cost. Natural therapy is not an overnight solution for restoration; it is more for prevention and maintenance, not emergencies. It will take time for your body to restore itself as you make changes. The perfect Vanilla Pound Cake bakes at 325 °F for one hour and 15 minutes. If baked at 450 °F for ten minutes, more than likely you will not have a perfectly baked cake. The same for natural healing, it takes time and patience to accomplish excellent health.

Nancy's Personal Space

Since we know that health is all about mindset, I believe that mental detoxification sets the foundation to a healthy lifestyle. We must learn to manage the stress and "stuff" that happens in our lives, to get to the real reason of why we cannot break those unhealthy habits, and how to resolve them. Expect setbacks with life transitions. The strategies here can prepare you to continue pushing forward. Several of my clients give excuses of why they cannot meditate or break bad habits, such as not having a quiet space in the house. For most, its' a lack of understanding the purpose of meditation, or skepticism about its benefits, but the number one reason is usually a lack of time.

Experts say most of us have a poor concept of time and how to manage it appropriately. During an experiment to determine a person's concept of actual time, they asked participants to keep their eyes closed for 60 seconds, relax and not count the seconds. When they thought that 60 seconds had elapsed, they were to quietly raise their hands. Most participants underestimated how much time had elapsed and raised their hands much earlier than 60 seconds. Generally, with better time management skills and with being intentional, we have more time to take care of ourselves.

Nancy had a million and one reasons why she could not complete this aspect of the program. Her number one reason was that she had no place in the house where she could spend time alone. Every room in the house had someone occupying it - children, children's friends and even grandchildren. After exploring her barriers, she finally came up with a solution; she found a small space on the floor of her closet and made it into a little sanctuary. I was very proud of her when she gave up the excuses and thought of a feasible solution to overcome this barrier. She placed her favorite blanket on the floor where she sat or laid, burned essential oils or incense and framed small pictures for inspirational thoughts. She made a do not disturb sign and placed it on the closed closet door during her meditation time. These things surrounded her in this tiny space during her meditation sessions. Now that she had a quiet place, she still found it difficult to find the time to meditate due to her busy schedule. I encouraged her to get up five minutes earlier and start with two minutes. She began to enjoy the process so much that she incrementally increased to ten minutes within two weeks. Nancy stated, "It allowed me to set my intentions for the day, pray and feel at peace during the day. I started the day relaxed and tranquility comes over me throughout the day." It also helped her to release some of her anxiety and daily stress and be more positive and intentional in her thoughts and actions. Nancy took control of her situation and stopped allowing circumstances to dictate her life choices.

Meditation does not always mean sitting still in a particular place. With practice and finding what style of meditation works for you, you can learn to meditate even while taking a shower or sitting in traffic.

Words of Affirmation

"You will be a failure, until you impress the subconscious with the conviction you are a success. This is done by making an affirmation that 'clicks'." - Florence Scovel Shinn

Daily positive affirmations are another form of mental cleansing and meditation. Repetition of anything becomes reality - that is the nature of the Universe. You must create the life you want by starting with your thoughts. There comes a point in time when we have to take responsibility for our destiny and stop blaming others, being stuck in the past or being content with the busyness of life. When life does not go the way we think it should or when "it" happens, habitually, we become bitter and fill our minds with negative thoughts and resentment. This allows the negative cycle of that karma to fester.

The next time you start to say negative things about yourself, or have negative thoughts, stop and think, "Is this something I would say to one of my kids or to a best friend?" Indeed, we have to learn to treat ourselves like our own best friend. We constantly hold onto past events due to guilt, shame, and unhealthy beliefs. For example, saying something such as, "My mother said I was stupid or I could never do anything right." Therefore, you tell yourself I am stupid, fat or ugly, and you allow these thoughts to dictate your present-day situation. I encourage you not to dwell on who wronged or hurt you, or any negative words spoken to you. Acknowledge this is not the situation right now, let it go and take steps for improvement.

Try it you, might like it

If you have never practiced meditation before, I encourage you to try it. Pick one of the modalities described below or find your own. If it is difficult for you, I encourage you to start slow; 2, 5, or 10 minutes 2-3 times a week and eventually work your way to at least 20 minutes daily and several short durations throughout the day. Initially, it can be very difficult to quiet the mind. As women, we face a great deal of pressure, we move through the day on automatic and it is difficult for us to push pause. We hit the ground running from the minute our eyes open in the morning and later have problems falling asleep.

During the meditation process, if you find it difficult to quiet your mind, it is usually best not to fight the thoughts. Let them come in and acknowledge them. Breathe into all that you are thinking and make a conscious decision to release it and move on without trying to resolve the issue at that moment. Do not get stuck on one thought for more than a few seconds. Once you learn to release your thoughts, you will begin to meditate anywhere, at work or in a midst of a crisis - all you need is a safe and peaceful space in your mind. Spending a few minutes each day in meditation, you begin to flow with life and manifest your desires with grace and ease.

Types of Meditation

Explore the various options and decide which one works best for you. Meditation can be very simple. Do not make it more difficult than it has to be. To learn more, there are many videos online, meetup groups in your area, or local yoga studios that offer free workshops on how to meditate. If you think you don't have time to learn how to meditate, or it's not important in this holistic approach, think about your life span, your future, your health, and give it a try it anyway. It is not difficult, once you get into the practice of it and make it your own, it becomes easier and you may find it to be a good "addictive" habit.

Six of the basic forms of meditation (there are many more option to explore):

Simple Meditation

This is one of the best meditation types for a beginner. It works great if you are not accustomed to sitting still for a period of time and focusing on your thoughts. It allows you to determine how much time you want to spend. Find a space that is peaceful - at your desk, in your car, in the restroom, in a closet, somewhere you can spend a few minutes in silence. Allow your mind to be still and think of nothing other than breathing, when a thought enters acknowledge it and let it go quickly, do not hold on to any particular thought. One of the challenges with this form of meditation is to focus on the task and not on how much time has passed. A great tool is an alarm. Setting an alarm discourages the brain from being preoccupied with how much time has passed. Set an alarm for the allotted time. Even if it's just one minute, once it goes off, the time is up and move on to the next task. Gradually, as you gain more control over your mind, your thoughts and senses, you will begin to increase the duration and explore other meditation techniques.

Transcendental Meditation

This is the most debated and researched form of meditation and, not to mention, it has become my favorite. Studies show this form of meditation helps in increasing intelligence and creativity. Some people have reported this form to be difficult because they fall asleep or nod off during the process. This can happen when the body becomes very relaxed. It is not necessary to master any particular type of breathing technique with this form of meditation. It is important to just inhale and exhale deeply while reciting a daily mantra consisting of encouraging words of inspiration that speaks to you. Such as "I am accepting a new job," "I have great friends," "I am prosperous." You're your statement in the present. It creates the opportunity and mindset that it's happening now. Whereas when you say, "I will have a new job," it puts it in the future and will usually feel out of reach. Focus on basic deep breathing and feeding oxygen to your body; focus on breathing in good health and breathing out the bad. This technique simply requires concentration by sitting in a relaxed posture, breathing, and releasing your thoughts.

Breath and Navel Meditation

This is the oldest technique recorded in China and India, and one of the most popular among other meditation types. It does require some form of controlled breathing technique. Sit in a relaxed posture and concentrate on your breath. A simple technique such as nostril breathing; in and out of the nostril is effective. Another is navel or abdomen breathing. Breathe in and expand the abdomen as much as possible, then exhale let the abdomen fall and let out all the air. Another technique is breathing through the nostril and breathing out with the mouth open.

Walking Meditation

Walking meditation involves focusing the mind on the feet while walking. When your mind wanders away from your steps, simply refocus it back to your steps and walking. This seems easy, but it can be challenging in practice. Time and patience makes it easier. It has proven to be a beneficial form of meditation and stress release.

Praying Meditation

Participate in a daily devotional. There are many books to help with this technique, including the Bible. Also, Joel Osteen has a wonderful book, *I Declare: 31 Promises to Speak Over Your Life*. John Maltby, a senior psychologist at Sheffield Hallam University, studied the effects of religion on the well-being of students. He found that, "Personal prayer was the most important factor, rather than simply being religious or attending services. The students who prayed suffered less from anxiety and depression."

One of my daily devotional is the Serenity Prayer: "...*Accept the things I cannot change; have the courage to change the things that I can; and the wisdom to know the difference."*

Body Scan or Grounding Meditation

Body scan meditation is very useful for people who have a difficult time falling asleep. You lie down and focus on your body parts; start from your toes to the hair on your head or reverse, but move in the direction just as an imagery x-ray. I practice this while falling asleep. Do not focus on your aches and pains or give reason to them; if something hurts, acknowledge it, release the pain and move on to the next body part and breathe good health or positive energy into it. This does not require a lengthy process. It can be as short or long a duration as you desire.

"We don't see things as they are…we see them as we are." - Anais Nin

Practical tips you can practice anytime and anywhere:

- Listen to nature sounds or inspirational music.
- If the weather is nice, get outside as much as possible and enjoy nature.
- Write your thoughts down on paper and review them.
- Stay positive. Adjust your attitude.
- Try deep breathing exercises. You can do this anywhere, while driving or sitting at your computer.
- Use essential oils, applying behind the ear or on your neck, temples or wrist. Be cautious when using topically; read the purchased brand's instructions before using. You can also use a diffuser. Some specific oils are great for stimulating the brain and relaxing: lavender, tea tree, eucalyptus, myrrh, frankincense, and peppermint are some of my favorites.

Thoughts to avoid because they can keep us in a negative state:

- Do you blame others for your stress? (i.e., boss, kids, spouse, coworkers)
- Do you define stress as a normal part of your life? (i.e., anxious, procrastinator, worry wart)
- Do you rationalize stress? (i.e., it's normal, necessary, or my responsibility)

"Nothing can stop a man with the right mental attitude from achieving his goal; nothing on earth can help a man with the wrong mental attitude." - Thomas Jefferson

Another one of my daily mantras that allows me to stay on track and make better choices: "I now take responsibility for making my life work. I respect my mind and body as God's temple, and give it only the best." The busier the external world, the more we need to cultivate stillness in the internal world. Reports show, 20 minutes of mental relaxation is the equivalent of two hours of sleep. Physical relaxation and mental clarity go hand in hand. Managing stress is all about taking charge of your thoughts, emotions, and perception.

SHOCKING FACT: Many people think it is selfish to take time out for themselves because it takes time away from the children or family. In actuality, if you do not take care of yourself, you may not be in a position to take care of others due to possible health concerns. Research shows that when parents do not take care of themselves or when they regularly talk about themselves in a negative manner, it gives their children a poor self-image and low confidence. It sends a message loud and clear: "I take care of others, but *not* myself."

Remember, happy kids come from happy parents. Not caring for yourself can reflect as a lack of self-love - please don't shoot the messenger. Regularly we end up creating the realities we most often fear because of the lack of control over our minds, which psychologists refer to as self-fulfilling prophecy or law of attraction. *"The discontent and frustration you feel is entirely your own creation,"* - Stephen Richards. If you desire the best health, act, speak, and meditate as if you are healthy, the behaviors will follow and become automatic. Eradicate negative talk and speak to yourself with confidence; believe in yourself and in your abilities.

CHAPTER 5

Good Night

"Think in the morning. Act in the noon. Eat in the evening. Sleep in the night." - William Blake

Cannot get out of bed? Do you wake up in a fog? Do you grab for coffee before you can do anything else? Are you tired all the time? Do you feel depressed? For thousands of people, falling asleep is not as simple as laying their head on a pillow. Most of us know the importance of sleep, but very few actually make it a habit to get the required amount of rest. Many of us not only have problems falling asleep, but also have trouble staying asleep. For the average person, when their head hits the pillow, this is the time their mind starts to wonder; everything that needs to get done and was not done comes to mind. We feel that life starts to close in around us, and we start to worry about everything, past, present, and/or future.

Due to its importance, sleep has been a hot topic for many years. Research shows that those who consistently sleep less than eight hours per night, typically have eating problems, weight issues, lack of energy, depression, skin conditions, premature aging, and other health concerns. The brain and body recovers and resets during sleep. A lack of sleep impacts the brain's function. Sleep deprivation has shown to decrease the immune system, lower melatonin (causing insomnia) and increases your health risk; it reduces productivity and efficiency, and has been blamed for many drowsy driving accidents. According to The Institute of Medicine, over one million injuries and between 50,000 and 100,000 deaths annually are results of preventable medical errors, many of which may have been the result of insufficient sleep. Doctors, especially newly graduated interns, are often expected to work continuous shifts of 24 to 36 hours with little or no opportunity for sleep.

Insufficient sleep can send our lives into a downward spiral ending with poor health. The unfortunate aspect of this is typically we do not attribute such concerns to something as basic as sleep. Many people have learned to function with less than the required amount on a regular basis, and we think that it is a normal way of life without realizing the harm that is being done to the nervous system. Refer to Chapters 3 and 4 for the importance of the nervous system. We depend on a burst of energy from coffee, energy drinks, and even prescription medication, all to end up feeling more drained, depleted, and eventually endangering the mind-body balance. There are herbs that have shown to help release stress and calm the mind (see Secret Five). This should only be used temporarily as it is not a permanent solution to creating better sleep habits.

Coffee, Tea or Sleep?

I spent many nights thinking of all the things that I needed to do the next day, what I forgot to do that day, was preoccupied with all my thoughts and life events, and could not fall asleep. Staying up late doing house work, catching up on paperwork or completing my homework assignments was a breeze because I could not sleep anyway; so, I might as well be productive with that time, or so I thought. This behavior continued for years; I thought it to be a badge of honor that I could stay up at night and function during the day. I did not realize that a lack of sleep was contributing to my poor eating habits, lack of energy, additional stress, diabetes, and skin and health problems.

I am not a coffee drinker, but I had my fair share of black tea and soda to give me that energy boost, which I should probably credit for my blood sugar issues - more on that in Secret Two. Many mornings, drinking a cup of black tea laced with white sugar and milk became more than just a childhood breakfast beverage; I needed it to give me a jolt of energy. Unfortunately, I felt tired, lacked energy and needed another boost before noon, so I turned to my favorite can of soda. The tea and soda pattern continued throughout the day. I did not think about the potential damage.

Hence, my system was probably too stimulated during the day, creating restless nights. I did not recognize the paradox I was caught in and how it would affect my long-term wellness. At the time, I did what I thought was best and what was an everyday "common" behavior for many others around me. I recalled driving home from work and nodding at the wheel frequently, due to fatigue and low blood sugar. When I started to experience symptoms of low blood sugar, I implemented some dietary changes, suggested by conventional practitioners but saw little results. I did not realize there were other factors I needed to implement to be successful, such as managing stress appropriately, decreasing tea and soda intake and getting more sleep.

Popular Demand

I began having health concerns prior to the Big D diagnosis, but healthcare professionals classified them as isolated incidents. Throughout my twenties and early thirties, I battled a severe case of Rosacea on my legs, arms and chest area for many years, alopecia (bald spots, not just thinning of the hair) and severe adult acne. As the years progressed, I became plagued with painful joints, muscle aches, constipation, digestive issues, and constant sickness with the cold or flu. Not once did a healthcare professional relate these issues to stress, unhealthy eating, or poor sleeping habits. The solution - pharmaceuticals - I used pharmaceutical treatments because I wanted a quick fix and did not believe there were other options for those ailments. At the time, I was not aware of the potential damages of the medications, even for short-term use. I took various medications for acne, rosacea, acid reflux and constipation. I had a few steroid treatments for alopecia and joint pain, all at various times over a three-year period with little improvement to my symptoms.

The life events I considered "normal" matters - poor dietary habits, abusive relationships, and motherhood - were being poorly managed and therefore, were causing sleep and health problems. Healthcare professionals were giving me accurate diagnosis of the problems, but still without real and permanent solutions for the root cause. I continued to get less than four hours of sleep on many nights; I took a nap during my lunch break and still needed to take a nap upon getting home from work before doing anything else.

Throughout the years, as I began this journey of holistic health, I identified various natural remedies, including supplements, which relieved some of the physical ailments. First, I stopped taking prescription medications. Initially, I had the mindset that if the natural remedies were working, why did I need to alter any of the physical behaviors, i.e. sleep (more on this in Secret Two). The common misconception is that since they're called supplements, it is acceptable to use long-term. It is just that - a supplement, not a permanent solution and not a means to an end (see Secret Five - Natural Healing).

Counting Sheep

Over the years, I did not consider replenishing and restoring energy through sleep, because the natural treatments seemed to remedy most of the symptoms. I finally conquered the soda addiction and incorporated other natural methods - acupuncture treatments for muscle and joint pain, vitamin D and other supplements, in which I experienced improvement with most of my symptoms. There was not enough time in the day to get everything done, so more sleep was not a priority. I thought as many of you probably think, "Sleep is something I can do later when I retire" and it really does not affect my health or how I function. A few years ago, my herbalist friend asked me to research the side effects of sleep deprivation. She speculated if I slept more, it would improve my sugar levels, acne, body pain and regular headaches, and put an end to the need for some of the supplements. I came across an article written by the Center for Disease Control, which stated, "Chronic Sleep Deprivation (CSD) has been tied to an increased risk of type 2 diabetes, cardiovascular disease, obesity, and depression." Considering that I averaged no more than 3-4 hours of sleep per night for several years, I was in that "chronic sleep deprived" category and showed symptoms to reflect that.

Getting to bed before 1:00 am was abnormal and proved to be very difficult for me. I tried methods suggested by experts like relaxation music and nature sounds, counting sheep, counting backward, a glass of wine before bed (probably the worst thing you can do), and a consistent bedtime, but still had trouble falling and staying asleep. Later, I realized while I implemented changes directly related to sleep habits, they were not very effective because I did not make changes to other aspects, such as my daily schedule or eating habits. I continued drinking caffeinated teas, stressing with a busy schedule and not meditating regularly; hence, the reason getting to bed earlier was not as effective, by itself.

Lastly, I discovered a few natural herbs that helped calm the mind and relax the body, such as Holy basil, Ashwagandha, Mother's Wort, St John's Wort, Rhodiala, L-Theanine and Valerian Root, which assisted me in falling asleep. I tried several of these at various times; Holy basil was my personal favorite. The effects of these supplements on the mind and nervous system vary from individual to individual. These herbs have multiple purposes and traditionally have shown to aid anxiety, boost immune system boosting, and balance hormones, to name a few of the benefits. After almost a year, I could not fall asleep without using one of these supplements. Sleeping should be a natural occurrence, but it was a challenge for me. It was time to make some other changes in my day to day routine.

Further research showed I also needed to change my dietary habits and implement stress management techniques as discussed in the previous chapter. It took almost a year before I could fall asleep and stay asleep without any type of natural sleep aid. Once I began to get an average of 6-8 hours on a consistent basis, I felt like a completely different person. Today, I have improved my sleep habits by 100% and take sleep very seriously. I am meditating on a regular basis and have learned to manage the stressors in my life. I limit watching murder, psychological mystery or dramatic movies or TV shows especially before bedtime. I surrounded myself with positive people and positive thoughts. In addition, I avoided caffeinated teas or drinks, sugary drinks/food, and managed what I ate. I have not taken prescription medication for anything in many years. Instead, I use herbal supplement for occasional restless nights, digestive problems and other concerns as they arise. It also helps to bring the body back in balance without much difficulty. I continue to stay abreast of new developments and make changes to assist in my natural health journey.

Sanctuary

In recent years, due to increased technology, we have been regularly exposed to electromagnetic frequencies, Wi-Fi, radio waves, microwaves, and x-rays that have been shown to deplete energy levels, increase hyperactivity, and possibly cause certain types of cancers and sleep disturbances. After much deliberation and a few years of convincing, John agreed to sell all but one television, including the one in our bedroom. We now maintain one TV in the living area; and to my surprise, he was on board with eliminating cable since we were not watching most of what TV had to offer.

We decided to treat our room as a sanctuary, only for sleep and sex; the kids were not allowed to play in our room. We removed the clock, radio, and television; unplugged the lamps and removed pictures of anyone other than John and me and that included the children and anything that resembled work, such as a desk. There are many studies on the importance of not having pictures of other people in your bedroom. They state that the imagery draws energy and allow you to think about the person(s) and any related issues, which keeps your mind in active mode. Therefore, it could attribute to your stress level and hinder falling asleep. I implemented wearing an eye mask to keep any natural lighting out. My cellular phone is the one electronic in the room and I keep it at a distance from the bed. I recorded inspirational words and prayer on a recorder and I listen to that before falling asleep. Implementing these changes over the years, I no longer use herbal sleep aids on a regular basis and I sleep an average of 7 hours per night.

It is still a challenge for me to physically get myself to the bed because I am a night owl and I work and think better at night. Due to being a night owl, I have to be intentional about bedtime or start my workday later to ensure adequate sleep. I set my phone alarm to alert me when it is time to begin bedtime preparation. It is tempting to ignore it at times, but I think back to the possible health consequence and falling back into bad habits, then it becomes effortless. When the alarm goes off, I honor myself and begin preparing for bed. Many times, it's easy to disregard the alarm or reminders, but honor your goals and intentions and get to bed. I like to have some down time or "me time" before falling asleep; simple things like brushing my teeth, taking a bath, reading for a few minutes, praying or meditating. Once in bed, regardless of what is going on in my life, I listen to my personal recording of inspirational message and I often fell asleep within 5 to 10 minutes. The inspirational messages I record are 15-25 minutes long. I change the message I listen to according to what is going on in my life and where I need meditation, inspiration, and prayer. Over the years as I have improved my sleep habits, I noticed I no longer suffered skin issues, fatigue, lack of energy or poor eating habits. I recognize my stressors and immediately do something about it because life does happen; it's a matter of how we prepare for it and what we do about it when it does.

What is Your Sleep Number?

Our body and brain uses sleep to recover from the daily grind. If you are physically active, you are not doing your body justice if you do not fully recover from the wear and tear. My clients often say, "I will rest when I am dead." I was one of those people who had that mentality. I thought it was admirable to be on the go constantly and did not believe sleep was important. Was I ever wrong and foolish to buy into that thought!

According to the National Sleep Foundation, recommended hours of sleep are:

- Newborns (0-3 mos.): Sleep range narrowed to 14-17 hours each day (previously it was 12-18)
- Infants (4-11 mos.): Sleep range widened two hours to 14-15 hours (previously it was 12-15)
- Toddlers (1-2 years): Sleep range widened by one hour to 12-14 hours (previously it was 11-14)
- Pre-schoolers (3-5): Sleep range widened by one hour to 11-13 hours (previously it was 10-13)
- School-age (6-13): Sleep range widened by one hour to 10-11 hours (previously it was 9-11)
- Teenagers (14-17): Sleep range widened by one hour to 8-10 hours (previously it was 8.5-9.5)
- Younger adults (18-25): Sleep range is 7-9 hours (new age category)
- Adults (26-64): Sleep range did not change and remains 7-9 hours
- Older adults (65+): Sleep range is 7-8 hours (new age category)

We know that sleep deprivation can contribute to poor health and can be responsible for early death. Studies show the amount of sleep needed varies from person to person, but there are a couple of factors consistent for most individuals: age and one's level of physical activity are the two main factors. The older and more physically active the person is, the more sleep is needed. Studies show that between the ages of 18-65 the average sleep requirement is 7-9 hours consecutively per night. If you're falling asleep, but awake throughout the night, it breaks the sleep pattern and you're basically starting all over again when you fall back to sleep. Therefore, the time does not constitute consecutive hours if you are awakened throughout the night.

Your Thoughts Have Meaning

"Your future begins with your next thought." - Bryant Mzy

Stress wreaks havoc on the central nervous system. Studies show that stress alone can cause sleep deprivation, increase in blood sugar levels, and the release of the hormone cortisol, which creates belly fat. Once you begin to recognize symptoms, it could be the beginning of many potential problems if you do not manage stressors.

Ephesians 3:20 tell us, *"Now to him who is able to do immeasurably more than we all ask or imagine, according to his power that is at work within us."* Many times, we get caught up and focus on at the negatives of our past, all the while selling ourselves short on what we have accomplished. Do not allow the stressor(s) in your life to cause you harm, because it will. High and constant stress is not good, as it can come at the cost of your health, relationships and sanity. Studies show that many people have experienced mental health illness such as bipolar, anxiety, Schizophrenia, and depression due to consistent, high levels of stress. It's important to learn how to handle both good and bad stress. When all else fails, stop, slow down and breathe. I have a saying, "I can't allow other people's problems to be my problem." This also pertains to adult children. If they get themselves into a pickle, help them resolve it, but do not take on their problems as your own or take responsibility for their thoughts, behaviors or consequences. This has taken me until recently to accept and put into action, but it helped calm my mind, once I did. We must become convinced that we are able to possess what God has promised us - good health, among many other things, and that helps to keep me on track.

Tips to Improve Your Sleep Lifestyle:

"You are what you think about all day long." - Dr. Wayne Dyer

Sleep should be a priority to managing stress, mental health, and maintaining a healthy lifestyle. There are daily habits, proven by research, of natural remedies to us help fall and stay asleep. It is not just our nighttime habits that we have to be mindful of, but also our behaviors during the day. Avoid the use of caffeine, coffee, cigarettes/tobacco, soda, energy drinks and sugary foods, particularly later in the day. These substances are enemies that can potentially damage organs, affect blood sugar levels, and contribute to sleep disturbances, which in turn can affect long-term health.

The tips provided below are those I wish I knew much earlier in life to help me sleep better and combat health concerns that led to taking prescription medication. I regularly implement many of these techniques and do not know how I ever slept before. Actually, I do know - I did not sleep. Many of these should be implemented, even if you do not have problems sleeping, in order to continue great health. When you release the mind and make better food choices, it can help you sleep better and the body recovers more efficiently.

- Establish a set bedtime. Get to bed at least 15-30 minutes earlier than the time you want to fall asleep.
- Establish a bedtime ritual. Practice deep breathing while doing a full body imagery relaxation - use essential oil i.e. lavender oil aromatherapy.

- The darker the room, the better. Use an eye mask or dark drapes. Darkness increases the hormone melatonin, which helps regulate sleep patterns and strengthen the immune system. Any form of light coming into your room can cause a decrease of melatonin over time, resulting in health issues.
- Reduce the environmental/external noise; use earplugs or white noise.
- Avoid using cigarette/tobacco, especially the closer you get to bedtime.
- Avoid sugary or caffeinated drinks and food throughout the day, especially in the evening. It's suggested to stop caffeine use at least 10 hours prior to bedtime.
- Eat healthy and nutritious balanced meals throughout the day. Stop eating large meals at least three hours prior to bedtime. This allows your body and metabolism to recover during sleep.
- Remove the television and other electronics from your bedroom. Avoid the use of any electronics at least one hour prior to going to sleep. Studies show that the blue light signals to the brain that it's daytime. Creating difficulty falling asleep.
- If possible, minimize electronic equipment close to the bed area, including radios and cell phones. Research shows that electrical items in your room cause energy to flow and can create brain stimulation, resulting in sleepless nights.
- Release your thoughts. Taking a warm Epsom Salt bath before bed is a great help in this regard, as it allows the body to detox. The magnesium from the Epsom Salts has been known to reduces stress, relax muscles and lower blood pressure.
- Spend some time reading or listening to relaxing music right before bedtime.
- Make your sleep space comfortable and pleasant.

- Respect the bedroom as your sleep zone and sanctuary. It is not a play area for the kids.
- Get regular exercise. Many studies have shown that people who work out later in the day sleep better. Exercising or walking increases endorphins, which reduces stress hormones. Therefore, you cannot use the excuse that it is too late to workout.
- If you have problems sleeping, avoid intensive physical activity at least two hours prior to bedtime. Instead, take a short slow walk before bedtime.
- Do not get out of the bed if you cannot fall asleep - that will only exacerbate the situation and makes it more difficult to fall asleep. Do not lay with your eyes closed hoping to fall asleep, instead do some light, leisure reading, and listen to relaxing sounds, music, or guided imagery.
- If you have a tendency to get up and use the restroom, make certain to empty the bladder before bed and avoid drinking anything at least 1 to 2 hours before bedtime.
- If you still have problems sleeping, literally turn your body upside down on the bed. Put your head at the foot of the bed and your feet at the head. If there is a headboard, prop your legs up and start deep breathing. Focus on your breath and give yourself permission to release your thoughts.
- Avoid hitting the snooze button when the alarm goes off in the morning. Set the clock for the latest possible time you allow yourself to sleep. When the alarm goes off, get up and out of the bed. Studies show that when you hit the snooze button and go back to sleep, you create a state of confusion in your brain. The brain is unable to decide if it's awake or asleep, and this causes you to wake up feeling even more foggy and tired than if you had gotten out of bed immediately without the snooze.

If you have tried any or all of these and they do not work, it is time to seek additional help. There are healthcare professionals who specialize in natural sleep therapy such as aggressive cognitive behavioral treatments/therapies that have proven to assist with falling and staying asleep without the use of pharmaceutical.

The key is discovering how to manage the stress life brings. We must change our perception of the current situation and not base it upon our pasts or our fears. Spend time alone. Meditate. Rest well. Our responsibility is to fear not! My mantra: "I will not fear sickness, disease, or plagues. I will not fear destruction or evil. I will not fear anything, for God is my refuge and my fortress, and He will deliver me." Positivity breeds positivity; negativity breeds negativity. If the mind is not in alignment, it is very difficult for our body to function optimally. If we are not dealing with stress appropriately, oftentimes it affects sleep patterns. If we do not get proper sleep, the body is not recovering and preparing to move forward. When the body is not prepared or recovered, it creates a trickle effect of other health problems over time. It is a dangerous roller coaster; it's crucial that you start to connect your mind-body.

"The world around you is a reflection of your inner world and how you perceive it." - Author Unknown

SHOCKING FACT: As a society, we are not managing life and stress appropriately. A Harvard Publication reported that over 264 million prescriptions were filled in 2011 for antidepressants - that only accounted for two of the most popular antidepressant medications and 23% of that number are women between the ages of 40-50. Are you taking care of your mind? By the time we go into a depressive state, stress has been piling on for a while and we are now in reactive mode. We must acknowledge the importance of caring for ourselves mentally, physically, and emotionally.

The tips and information given here are lifestyle changes; they are not something to do once and forget. These techniques must be built into our daily routine in order to balance the mind-body connection and to promote a healthy nervous system. Life will bring stress - it is simply up to you to ensure that you deal with it properly. I keep this poem at my desk to help stay on track when I falter.

Think Positive
by Walter D. Wintle

If you THINK you are beaten, you are

If you THINK you dare not, you don't

If you like to win, but you think you can't
It is almost certain you won't.

If you THINK you'll lose, you're lost.

For out of the world we find,
Success begins with a fellow's will.

It's all in the state of mind.

If you THINK you are outclassed, you are.

You've got to THINK high to rise,
You've got to be sure of yourself before
You can ever win a prize.

Life's battles don't always go
To the stronger or faster man,
But sooner or later the man who wins

Is the man who THINKS he can!

CHAPTER 6

Secret Two: Food for Life

"Toxic" Dinner

"When we are motivated by goals that have deep meaning, by dreams that need completion, by pure love that needs expressing, then, we truly live life."

- Greg Anderson

Throughout the world, major shifts in dietary patterns are occurring, even in the consumption of basic products, towards creating more options, variety, and more diversified diets. Many of these changes are due to the increase of the world's population and demand on the food industry. John Kearney, author and researcher at The School of Biological Sciences, Dublin Institute of Technology, also attributes it to factors including urbanization and food industry marketing. The policies of trade liberalization over the past two decades have implications for health by virtue of being a factor in facilitating the 'nutrition transition' that is associated with rising rates of obesity and chronic diseases such as cardiovascular disease and cancer.

In most recent years, we have seen a shift in the quality of food. Although there are more organic, Non-GMO (genetically modified organism) and natural (no antibiotics, no hormones etc.) food alternatives available, the number of Americans eating processed food and fast food continues to increase each year. I was astonished by the amount of money the average household spends on processed food and fast food. Research shows most American households spend 90% of their grocery budget on processed food, fast food, and unhealthy snacks. Based on a study done by National Public Radio, as of 2012 Americans now spend 22.9% of their household budget on processed food, which includes frozen dinners, canned soups and sugary snacks. This is an increase of 11.6% since 1982. One of the key principles to achieving better health is to ensure the majority of food consumption is all natural, organic, fresh, chemical free and locally grown when possible. It should be low in artificial preservatives, sugar and salt.

Like many Americans, your diet may be comprised of more than the occasional deli meat. It probably includes other processed food such as soda, cookies, canned soup, and potato chips, which contain thousands of potentially harmful chemicals. National Health Services (NHS) defines processed foods as, "Foods that aren't just microwave meals and other ready meals. The term 'processed food' applies to any food that has been altered from its natural state in some way, either for safety reasons or convenience." Most processed foods have some form of added salt, sweeteners, fat, preservatives and other ingredients. The added ingredients in these basic foods extend the shelf life, adds flavor and are inexpensive, yet it could be costing us our health. This includes breakfast cereals, frozen meals, cheese, canned vegetables, bread, potato chips, bacon, oils, milk and deli meat. As typical consumers, we do not consider how these added ingredients may be affecting our overall wellness, possibly contributing to weight gain, hormonal issues, inflammation, high blood pressure, high cholesterol, diabetes and digestive issues, among many other ailments.

It is important to point out that not all processed foods are unhealthy. Some foods, such as oil, and milk, need to be processed to make them safe to consume, while canned produce and deli meat may have added salt, sweeteners and other chemicals, which makes them unhealthy. Frozen fruits and vegetables without added ingredients contain more vitamins and nutrients than canned. Err on the side of caution, read the ingredients and nutritional labels on any product. Those added ingredients could be harmful to your health. It's best to know what is in the food you are eating.

Pharmaceuticals or Food?

I have managed diabetes without pharmaceuticals or direct assistance from "traditional" healthcare providers. When given my diagnosis, they did not offer me much assistance other than medication, which I was not willing to take it. When my physician said, "Good luck with that," after I refused pharmaceuticals, I could not necessarily blame him. More than likely, he probably perceived prescription medication as the only or best treatment option available. It is likely that most of his patients accepted the medication and a large percentage would never stop using it. This is usually due to the lack of knowledge and understanding that diabetes can be reversed in many cases, through diet and exercise.

While in the doctor's office, my intuition said there had to be another - and maybe better - solution than medication. At that moment, I had no idea reversal was possible. My previous experience with taking pharmaceuticals for other health concerns did not resolve the problem, so I knew it was not an option for me the time. When I asked my physician if it was something that would eventually resolve, he said, "No, this is something you will have for the rest of your life, and in order to control it, you must take the medication." The information I used to reverse diabetes, and am sharing here, I learned through non-traditional means. I had family members die prematurely from complications of diabetes while using pharmaceuticals. After witnessing what family members went through and still died, it was a no-brainer for me. At the time, the only thing I was aware of that could possibly mitigate the situation was to limit my candy, soda, and pastry intake. Educating myself about diabetes became a priority; controlling it with food, exercise, and reducing stress was a foreign concept.

When I started this journey and began researching, the Internet was not fully accessible, which meant spending many hours at the library, bookstores, and in classes to learn the ins and outs of this illness and develop a course of action to resolve it. It felt as if I was in college all over again, as I spent numerous hours researching and gathering information. Eager for knowledge, I asked questions to anyone who was willing to talk and I spoke with many nutritionists and dietitians. The information they shared was heavily influenced by conventional medicine, such as: limiting soda, carbohydrates, and candy/chocolate; drinking orange juice each morning to regulate and stabilize my sugar levels; eating wheat bread instead of white bread; and eating brown rice instead of white rice.

Those dietary changes were implemented and no improvements were noted. I was still very dependent on glucose tablets and peppermint candy to get me through most days when I experienced the hypoglycemic phase. Orange juice only made matters worse; shortly after drinking it, my sugar levels dipped significantly. I will explain later in the book why that was not the best alternative. I started a food journal to record what I was eating and how it affected my sugar levels. It was very time consuming, tedious and sometimes not always consistent, but, in retrospect, I am glad I did it. It was time well spent, and it possibly saved my life.

Alternative Medicine is an Option

During my continued research, I came across information about alternative medicine - using food, herbs, and supplements to heal the body. I set out to find an herbalist, naturopathic practitioner and/or natural health advisor in my area. They were rare at that time, and when I did find one within a reasonable distance, the cost of an average visit was roughly $350 per hour. That was more than my social worker budget could afford and medical insurance did not cover any portion. Suffice it to say, I was disappointed to find myself back to square one and unable to engage the assistance of one of these healthcare professionals. I would not have given up so easily if I knew then what I know now. I would have begged, borrowed, and done anything to be able to have a person practicing natural alternative medicine to help me through the process. It would have made my life 100% easier, saving me the time, frustration and money in the long run,

As I often say, everything happens for a reason and in its Divine time. If I did not have to take this difficult journey and learn by experimentation, I may not be able to share this space with you now. I had to become my biggest advocate and "doctor" in order to reverse this disease and put myself in a proactive state to resist other diseases. The more I researched, the more amazed I became at how conventional healthcare professionals were uninformed about alternative health care. I became adamant and was convinced that I could reverse diabetes without medication. I had to figure out how to put the pieces together to make it work properly.

A couple of years had gone by since my diagnosis and I started to wean myself off the junk food and soda addiction, avoiding these items at all costs. I occasionally ate fast foods, frozen meals, boxed, and canned food. At the time, I did not find any solid evidence that said it wasn't healthy, nor did I realize the effects the artificial ingredients had on my sugar level. I rationalized with myself that I would continue to use these products out of convenience and they weren't necessarily bad for me.

I started to incorporate things I learned and some of them worked for me, such as eating small balanced meals every 2-3 hours, increasing protein intake, and eliminating candy bars and sodas for lunch was no longer my norm. When I made those small changes, the hypoglycemic episodes decreased. Honestly, I thought even if I could decrease the occurrences of my unstable sugar levels, it would put me into a safe zone. Little did I know I was still damaging my health by continuing to eat fast, processed, and comfort foods, not enough fruit and vegetables, and was not appropriately managing the stressors in my life. I was having relationship issues, relocating to a different state, starting a new job that was not working out, financial issues, all while being a single parent. Therefore, I was still eating emotionally and foolishly endangering my health; I did not believe the numbers (sugar levels) were important. I determined my health according to how I felt every day. As long as I was not experiencing any physical symptoms, I thought all was well.

Convenience of Processed Food

I started to limit my fast food intake, not for health, but for financial reasons. I realized I was spending a large chunk of my budget eating out, particularly for lunch during the weekday. I was saving to buy my first house, on a social worker's salary, while solely being financially responsible for my daughter, and graduate school expenses. My exorbitant food costs were no help. As a result, I became dependent on the next best thing, frozen dinners, canned and boxed meals. They were delicious, quick, and easy to make. They got me out of the kitchen fast and provided me with a great meal, or so I thought.

As a busy single mom, working and attending graduate school, I did not think giving up processed foods would be easy. I thought cooking homemade meals would make my schedule more hectic, because it was time consuming, especially since cooking was NOT my forte. In order to save money, I avoided eating restaurant fast food, but ate other processed foods that were affordable and easy to prepare. Things I could grab and go - frozen, boxed, and canned meals. I was unaware of the ingredients in these foods that were probably adding to my health issues and causing my daughter to become sick, as well. My diabetic symptoms were still unstable; my daughter and I had periodic stomachaches, frequent colds and flu, and occasional ear infections. I started to experience severe acne, hair loss, and rosacea; even then, I thought those were normal health struggles and I did not make many modifications.

Read the Ingredients List

"Take care of your body. It's the only place you have to live." - Jim Rohn

It was difficult for me to give up the convenience of processed food due to my stressful lifestyle, emotional eating and pure habit. Eating better can be frustrating because of all the options at our disposal. Today, there are many healthier options available and more reasonably priced than in previous years. Changes are being made every day to our food, and some manufacturers are finding ways to make unhealthy food appear healthy by putting deceiving labels on products. A label may say, "sugar free" while there are added artificial sweeteners. In the case of the word "natural" on labels - a certain amount of pesticide, hormones or antibiotics is permitted without having to state it on the label. It is difficult to know all the harmful ingredients unless you are an expert in the field or it's your full-time job.

A rule of thumb: If you buy canned food, frozen meals, pre-packaged items, even bottled water, read the ingredients list carefully. Look for the ones with the least number of additives, preservatives and ingredients, non-GMO and organic. If there are words you do not recognize, cannot pronounce, or the list includes more than five ingredients, it's something you probably want to avoid or limit.

Recent reports are linking consistent use of processed food to unhealthy habits and emotional eating. These foods can become addictive due to their high sugar and salt content. Three facts about unhealthy eating and processed food were consistently repeated in the reports:

1. Avoid canned, pre-packaged meals or frozen dinners.
2. Avoid or limit dairy intake.

3. Avoid and limit simple sugars, artificial sweeteners and simple carbohydrates.

Sounds easy, but it's not. I will not tell you it will take 7 days, 21 days or even 28 days to eat healthier food, stop the cravings, develop time management skills, or break emotional eating. According to a recent study published in the European Journal of Social Psychology, a daily action like eating fruit at lunch or running for 15 minutes took an average of 66 days to become a habit. Forming new habits takes time; establishing intentional behaviors and mindset shift takes practice and maybe some help from a health advisor or coach. Be patient with yourself, move forward and make constant incremental improvement. A simple step to get started - decide which of the three unhealthy habits listed in the steps above you want to work on first, and then go for it. There are many ways to eat better. If you stick to some of the basics given here, it could have a profound impact on your eating habits and ultimately, your health.

Here are some examples of processed foods to avoid:

Frozen meals, canned fruit, and vegetables; most deli meats and bacon; most breads; most packaged snacks: dried fruit and vegetable, chips, granola bars; flavored nuts; microwave popcorn, ice cream; most soft drinks and carbonated drinks; most condiments - ketchup, mustard, barbeque sauce, spaghetti sauce; and milk. These are all foods that, over time, should be avoided or limited for better health. This is, of course, if you want to lose weight, reverse diabetes, skin problems, infections, and other health concerns.

Here are some examples of ingredients found in processed and other food items that should be avoided or limited.

Ingredients to AVOID/LIMIT

- Sodium nitrite (causes cancer)
- MSG / monosodium glutamate / yeast extract (causes obesity and nerve damage)

- Hydrogenated oils (causes heart disease)
- High-fructose corn syrup / sugar / sucrose (causes diabetes and obesity)
- Artificial colors (causes behavioral disorders)
- Artificial Sweeteners; Aspartame (causes brain damage, kidney failure, optic nerve damage)
- Homogenized milk fats (causes heart disease and cardiovascular disorders)
- Red meat (absolutely no beef, pork, or other red meat)
- Cow's milk, cheese and dairy products
- Soft drinks, junk foods, snack foods or fast foods
- Processed foods such as cookies, crackers, and frozen dinners
- Fried foods
- Fruit juice drinks and flavored bottled water
- White flour and any foods containing white flour
- Refined carbohydrates such as breads, cereals, pastries, and pizza dough

SHOCKING FACT: Processed foods are not a modern convenience - they have been around since the first barrel of salt-pork sailed across the Atlantic in the 17th century. These foods provide convenience and give us access to foods that would otherwise perish in transit. It is recommended that if you enjoy these foods, eat them in moderation and use common sense. Check the nutrition labels to avoid anything high in fats, sugars, salt and chemicals you cannot pronounce. Be sure to make fresh, simple ingredients the focus of your lifestyle.

In order for this epidemic to change, each individual must change their eating habits and be cognizant of the food and other products we purchase. We must step up and advocate for future food policies to consider both agricultural and health sectors, and overall food that is more nutritious. This would enable the development of reasonable and sustainable policies, ultimately benefitting agriculture, human health, and the environment. We must take a stand in what we subject our families and ourselves to by being mindful of the food and household products we bring into our homes.

Limit or avoid these household products due to potential harsh ingredients. This is not the case for every brand, hence the importance of reading the content/ingredient list.

- Popular-name laundry detergents (loaded with toxic fragrance and petroleum-based chemicals)
- Popular deodorants and antiperspirant (contains aluminum and sulfate)
- Toothpaste and mouthwash (may contain fluoride)
- Popular shampoos / soaps / conditioners (all contain harmful fragrance chemicals)
- Dryer sheets (contain fragrance chemicals)
- Air and Carpet Fresheners (contain fragrance chemicals)
- Perfumes/Cologne

CHAPTER 7

The "Art" of Cooking

"I don't like food that's too carefully arranged; it makes me think that the chef is spending too much time arranging and not enough time cooking. If I wanted a picture, I'd buy a painting." - Andy Rooney

Cooking 101

With an increase of stressful events and life responsibilities, we find ways to make life a little more convenient. Too often, there is not enough time left to cook a meal after coming home from work. Instead, we choose fast food restaurants, pizza, frozen or microwavable meals, canned or boxed food. It is unrealistic to expect a three-course meal to be served every night, but you should make an effort to cook a basic, non-processed meal, i.e. homemade soup, stir-fry, or a meatloaf for you and your family. The bottom line is when it comes down to your health, nothing is superior to eating the most natural, unprocessed foods prepared in your kitchen.

According to research by Johns Hopkins Bloomberg School of Public Health, people who frequently cook meals at home eat healthier and consume fewer calories than those who do not. There are many benefits to cooking at home using raw ingredients - you save money and time, use less salt, sugar, artificial sweeteners, trans fats, and consume less calories. When we cook healthier meals at home, we tend to eat a more balanced and nutritious meal, to include protein, complex carbs, and unsaturated fats. Researchers found that 8% of adults cooked dinner once or less a week. This same group consumed, on an average day, 2,301 total calories, 84 grams of fat, and 135 grams of sugar. Whereas 48% of participants who cooked dinner 6-7 times a week consumed 2,164 calories, 81 grams of fat and 119 grams of sugar in a typical day.

Having a balanced meal and using less processed food allows the body to feel satisfied, thus you eat less calories and experience fewer cravings. Other benefits may include fewer chemicals ingested, fewer doctor visits, more energy, quality family time, weight control and eating smaller portions. Getting a grasp of your weight and wellness is reason alone to start cooking at home and eating a healthier diet. Obesity is a symptom to a much larger issue. "Obesity is an escalating public health problem that contributes to other serious health issues, including diabetes, high blood pressure, and heart disease," says Wolfson, a researcher at Johns Hopkins.

To Grandma's House We Go

How to cook or begin to cook is not a one-size-fits-all solution. I completely understand that time and financial constraints may be considered barriers to healthy cooking, and frequent cooking may not be feasible for everyone. However, for most individuals, once you learn the "art of cooking" it becomes simple and you begin to wonder why you did not do it more often or at all. I had to figure out how to cut my food expense to save money. I tried limiting fast food and eating out, but that was not enough. While eating frozen and processed meals helped with the budget, physically, we were experiencing headaches, acne, weight gain, stomachache, colds, unstable blood sugar, and a lack of energy. My initial efforts to wean off processed food were not because I was aware of the potential dangers; it was to save money. At the time, I found very little information on and was oblivious to toxins in our food and how they related to many health issues. It was just by happenstance that I saw a positive change in my family's and my overall well-being, when I began preparing home-cooked meals and eating at my mom's.

Initially, I thought processed and fast foods were the least expensive route, but after taking a closer look at how much money I was spending on "food" and medical bills, I had to rethink this strategy. In order to save money, I had to avoid eating out and using the "easy foods." That meant I had to learn to cook from scratch, semi-scratch, or go to my mother's house more often to eat. How was I to start cooking non-canned or boxed meals, I didn't know how or where to start? I could not boil an egg or cook rice without burning it. I tried cookbooks, but the meals tasted awful and took more than the hour I had allotted to prepare it. I did not have an extra 1-2 hours every day to spend in the kitchen.

My mother, an experienced and excellent cook, spent an average of 45 minutes to an hour to prepare a meal. My impression of cooking was time-consuming, difficult, and required a certain skill I did not possess; therefore, it did not seem like a viable option for me. My options were either to continue eating the processed food and getting sick, learn how to cook, or go to my mother's house. The latter seemed to be a more viable option since the others were not working to my advantage. I started to eat more often at my mother's house – which was not a permanent solution.

Last Alternative

I looked for and tried every other possible option before resorting to "home" cooking. I even tried to get my mother to cook at my house, but she graciously declined. I tried several cookbooks, including a popular "semi-homemade" cookbook, without much success. Taking cooking classes or hiring a personal chef was my next thought but it was not financially feasible. In the mid-90s downloading a YouTube video or a recipe was not an option as such technology did not exist at the time. Finally, I asked my mother for help and she was thankful I finally had a desire to cook, after years of trying to convince me of the benefits. My mother came over a couple days a week for hands-on guidance and to answer questions. We put together simple and quick meals. I had a busy life, so the last thing I needed was to spend hours in the kitchen after a long day at work and graduate school. I believed making home cooked meals would help me save money, and it did. A pack of chicken cost about $.99 cents per pound - those were the days - which gave me 3-4 servings compared to one serving of a frozen dinner for $1.00. Commonly, we think it's impossible to eat healthy on a budget, but that's an absolute misconception. Regardless of your budget constraints, work/school schedule, or family size, you can enjoy healthy food at a low cost.

Cooking Made Simple

For starters we made simple meals like broiled chicken, fried catfish, broiled pork chops, grilled steaks, red beans and rice, steamed broccoli, sautéed spinach, corn on the cob and mashed potatoes. I made big batches so we would have enough leftovers to take for lunch and two nights of dinner. I could not believe I was cooking! It did not taste quite like mom's, but it was decent. I mastered these items and stuck with them for many years, adding a few other items such as spaghetti and tuna casserole along the way. My daughter recently had a conversation with a friend about their favorite childhood foods. My daughter said, "All I remembered eating as a kid was catfish, red beans, and rice." We laughed so hard, acknowledging how far I had come with my cooking ability.

Occasionally, I used canned beans and boxed items like mac and cheese, hamburger helper and Tuna Helper, some of my daughter's favorite - it was a start, right? Initially, I began home cooking to help with my budget, and stuck with it because I liked the impact it had on my savings account and positive changes in our health. It is only within recent years that I learned the dangers of processed and fast foods and that, unbeknownst to me, I was saving our health and, ultimately, our lives.

"The roots of education are bitter, but the fruit is sweet." - Aristotle

Cooking 101: Here are some practical tips to help you get started. These tips can save your life, and allow you to save more for that vacation, to buy a house, or for your retirement (think big).

1. Ask for help from a friend, family member, or me.
2. Attend cooking classes or hire me or another menu preparation coach
3. Find simple recipes online (don't be afraid to alter them to your taste or find alternative "healthier" ingredients). For example, instead of regular flour, use coconut flour. Find oil alternatives like olive, coconut, or grapeseed oil.
4. Make it simple: Broiled chicken/fish; brown or wild rice; roasted, baked, or mashed red or sweet potatoes; steamed broccoli; carrots; roasted Brussels sprouts.
5. Watch my YouTube channel.
6. Download recipes from YouTube, Pinterest, Allrecipes.com, Foodnetwork.com, etc.
7. Make cooking a social event - cook with friends
8. Make a grocery list and stick to it.
9. Try making at least 2-3 meals a week for 90 days. Take note of the changes and see how you feel.

One of the many advantage to cooking your own meal is that you know exactly what is in it. Remember my childhood story: We ate all-natural meats, fruit and vegetables directly from our backyard, and made homemade meals and desserts. Yet, my grandmother still suffered from diabetes. Why was this? Keep in mind that even with homemade foods, we tend to still use processed items like white sugar, deli meat, bacon, iodized salt, white flour, margarine, canned tomatoes, ketchup, milk, lard, fructose and/or corn syrup, artificial color, artificial sweeteners and hydrogenated this and that. Therefore, it is of the utmost importance to pay attention to the ingredients you are using when making "healthier" home-cooked meals, treats, or snacks.

SHOCKING FACT: Does eating every 2-3 hours matter? The purpose of cooking at home was to initially save money, but we benefited in many other ways; having home cooked food readily available decreased my chance of eating unhealthy and encouraged me to eat regularly. Studies also show that a huge aspect of weight loss and disease management is NOT STARVING (more on this in Chapter 8). Reports show that healthy eating is "at least 80% of the challenge and 70% of weight loss is WHEN, WHAT, and WHY you eat." Eating regularly increases metabolism, boosts nutrients, decreases cravings, and contributes to weight loss.

CHAPTER 8

God's Gracious Gift

"Cooking is not difficult. Everyone has taste, even if they don't realize it. Even if you're not a great chef, there's nothing to stop you from understanding the difference between what tastes good and what doesn't."

- Gerard Depardieu

The top reasons most people say they do not cook are lack of cooking skills and not enough time. Yet, studies show that Americans spend more time watching the Food Network channel than actually preparing their own meals. Over time, as a society, we have allowed the food industry to fatten us and weaken quality family ties, creating a displacement of home cooked meals and more microwavable options. In 1900, 2% of meals were eaten outside the home. In 2010, 58% of meals were eaten away from home, with one in five breakfasts from McDonald's.

Recent studies show this current generation will have the shortest life span of the last 100 years. There is no argument that society has changed because there are more couples and mothers working outside the home full-time, more latchkey kids now than ever before, and advanced technology is more accessible with more options available at rapid speeds. We cannot continue to allow society to change the values within our home. We are raising a generation that is preoccupied with technology, instant gratification and self-absorbed, glorified social media lifestyles; yet, their self-esteem continues to decrease while the suicide rate increases.

As a nation, we have become slaves to our careers, jobs, and social media. Families are not spending enough quality time together. Most family meals occur about three times a week, last less than twenty minutes, and are spent watching television or texting while each family member eats a different microwave meal. We eat more meals in the car than the kitchen. The importance of what we are teaching our children and what we put on our table has never been more imperative. The earth will survive our self-destruction, but we may not. Years of scientific research has proven the only way to obtain good health is by being intentional about what we put into our bodies: real, whole, local (if available), fresh, unprocessed, foods free of chemical, hormone and antibiotics.

My Personal Chef

When I met my husband, John, I was still making my specialty of mashed potatoes, broccoli, catfish, broiled chicken, and spaghetti. He began cooking because he was much better at it and more health conscious. My daughter loved the change from my insipid cooking she endured for years. John was what most people, including me at the time, referred to as a "health nut." Initially, I thought, "What did I get myself into?" He did not eat beef, pork, most dairy products or fried food. He avoided the use of cheese, sour cream, oil or butter, yet his meals had the taste of a gourmet chef. I was still discovering and working to simplify my healthier lifestyle and was open to his dietary habits.

John made cooking seem simple and effortless. I initially felt intimidated to be in the kitchen with him. The only canned items he occasionally used were canned beans or tomatoes; he avoided all frozen and boxed meals. He began eating healthier about five years prior to meeting me and was not changing his eating habits.

I thought I knew a thing or two about healthy eating; John's wellness habits were on a higher level. What I thought was healthy did not compare to his lifestyle. He worked out 6-7 days per week, including recreational basketball and football. He ate things such as egg whites only (not the best idea, more about this later), chicken and turkey (white meat only), fish, steamed vegetables, occasional skim milk, and many carbohydrates. Later, we will discuss why some of what he thought was healthy was actually not. In the beginning, I thought I would die of starvation because of the new lifestyle he had introduced, not because the food was bad, but I just could not fathom preparing one of his meals.

I recall the first meal John prepared when we started dating. It was baked chicken stuffed with spinach and crabmeat, with a homemade non-dairy cream of mushroom sauce, and garlic-mashed potatoes. He used no butter or milk. My daughter and I looked at each other and said, "OMG!" That is really an understatement of our reaction. Mashed potatoes loaded with butter were her favorite and she was not aware that he didn't use butter in the mashed potatoes and could not tell the difference. We thought we were at a four-star restaurant. We both said, "Ma's (my mother) cooking is good, but not like this." My internal light bulb was turned on by this cooking episode, and I realized that those fancy meals at restaurants *could* be duplicated at home, effortlessly. This was better than the restaurant, because he did not use all the bad oils, cream, and salt that they probably would have. It gave me a real glimpse at healthy cooking made simple. John is not a trained chef – he simply learned how to do these things by trial and error and having a passion for real food. He knew what he liked and how he wanted it to taste and that was his foundation for cooking.

The Worst Gift a Man Gives a Woman

During the first few years of our marriage, John did most of the cooking, and I did not have a problem with it. He was a much better cook than I. He made all the foods we enjoyed, with a healthy twist. It was great to get out of the kitchen and take that load off my shoulders. Over time and due to his demanding work schedule, cooking became less of a priority and very taxing for him. He tried to get me in the kitchen, but I really did not want that full-time job back. As a compromise, we agreed to alternate weeks, which allowed us both a break, but it did not take away the dreaded feeling I had of cooking, which increased his anxiety level.

I knew I had to remain on this path if I wanted to continue with significant improvements in my health as I had seen in the last few years. Many of my symptoms - constant urination, low blood sugar crashes, passing out, dry mouth, leg cramps, acne, colds and flu, had been non-existent since John took over the kitchen. If I wanted to continue to live a life I felt I deserved without being sick, home cooking, use of non-processed ingredients and healthier food was the best option. Sometimes I resorted to old habits and had processed and/or fast food, because it was quick and easy, but John refused to eat it and therefore, he was back in the kitchen preparing his own meals. It was unfair to him to come home and cook after working long hours. That meant I had to make a fervent effort to cook according to his healthier style. I also noticed that with my style of cooking, within a short period, some health concerns began to reoccur.

When I cooked, I rarely included vegetables, and added a lot of simple carbohydrates along with some processed items. I recall venturing out and preparing a vegetable soup. Although the recipe called for many vegetables I had never eaten, I was willing to try. The soup included Brussels sprouts, green peas, green beans, cauliflower and leeks, and it looked delectable. The broth was delicious, but I could not eat the vegetables as it literally made me gag. On the contrary, John and mother said it was one of the best vegetable soups. My daughter and I tried to eat it, but considering we did not like many vegetables, we could not eat something we did not enjoy. I knew the health benefits of eating vegetables, but I just did not have an acquired taste for them.

One year for my birthday, John gave the one gift most women dread getting and men should avoid giving - a household item. He gave me a Vitamix and I was livid. Livid was an understatement! I was expecting jewelry or a handbag - I could not believe he gave me a kitchen item as a birthday present. When he saw the look on my face, he said, "This blender was expensive and I thought it would be a great present. You need to acquire a taste for and increase your vegetable intake." He thought blending vegetables would be easier for me to ingest. Thus, inspiring me to try more of a variety, to increase greater health and at least consume the recommended daily amount, which I was not getting regularly.

He had good intentions, but I was still upset because it involved the kitchen item - but I kept it just to appease him. It came with a recipe book that not only included vegetable smoothies, but fruit smoothies, popsicles, ice cream, and soup; all of my favorites. I love to eat, but cannot eat anything I do not enjoy. It must be tasty and appealing or I will not eat it regardless of the health benefits. I decided to make a few of the vegetable and fruit smoothies, soup and ice cream recipes. Initially, in order to drink the vegetable smoothie, I added more fruit than the recipe called for to make it more flavorful, but I still held my nose and drank as fast as possible.

Eventually, my taste buds adapted and after many months, it became tolerable to ingest. As my taste buds changed, I took away some fruit and introduced a variety of vegetables. I started with a few ingredients, Brussels sprouts, radish, leeks, kale, asparagus, and beets and incorporated other combinations over time. I had never eaten those vegetables before using the Vitamix. As much as I hated to admit it, my husband was right. Using the blender allowed me to increase my vegetable intake by 100% and acquire the taste for new vegetables. Now, 13 years later, I eat many of those vegetables raw and cooked on a daily basis. We still have the Vitamix - it's one of the best presents.

The Aha! Moment

One day during a conversation, John said, "I noticed you haven't had many blood sugar episodes or tested your sugar levels within the last few months." As I thought about it, he was right. The only thing we could attribute it to, was *how and what* I was eating, reducing my stress levels, and being more physically active. We were both cognizant of making healthier changes as the years progressed and new research developed. As John's job continued to become more demanding and called for him to work later hours, it made it difficult for him to cook every other week. I had a choice to make; either prepare home cooked, "healthy" meals and having control over my family's and my health concerns, or return to processed and fast food. If I chose the latter, I would have to be prepared to encounter vision problems, skin conditions, mood swings, tingling in my legs, and low energy.

I developed a new respect and appreciation for the mindset, rather than the art of cooking. I made a mindset change. I embraced the idea that if I continued to improve my eating and lifestyle habits, my health would continue to improve as well. This could not be a week or month long *diet* or change. It came with time, and it had to be permanent in order for me to experience long-term effects. That meant I had to find enjoyable ways to eat, think, and feel; this was not something I learned from books or classes, but from trial and error and my personal struggles on this journey to live healthier. And healthier we became.

The first time I went with John to his annual physical, the doctor was amazed with his blood panel - heart rate and blood pressure results. He called the nurses into the office to show them what a "true cholesterol level" looked like. "I don't see many people as healthy as you," the doctor said. When I heard that, I was even more convinced that I had to change if I wanted to live a healthier lifestyle - with "healthier" cooking and a better choice of foods being a huge part of that equation. As I began to incorporate some of his healthy habits with what I had researched and learned, I began to live a life without worrying about passing out, and felt that I was actively working to extend my life, and improve the way I look and feel.

Changing our eating habits did not mean eating things we did not enjoy, eating bland food, depriving ourselves of what many call "the good stuff," having fun, eating passionately, or drinking alcohol. It meant being aware, being intentional, and trying a variety of food items. I had to love our lives enough to make small sacrifices for longevity. We had "treat foods" in moderation and used healthy alternative ingredients. It also meant respecting the life and body that God blessed me with, and choosing to live life abundantly. I realized by changing how and what I ate, how I treated my mind and spirit, it was realistic to live without headaches, joint pain, lethargy, blurry vision, dizziness, nausea and passing out.

I loved the health advantages I encountered from home cooked meals and blending raw vegetables. I felt energized and worked out 3-4 days a week. My hair was growing long and thick, and the acne cleared up; headaches and anxiety dissipated; hypoglycemic episodes had decreased and blood sugar levels were consistently normal. My daughter's episodes of colds and ear infections reduced drastically. Yet, I still did not like slaving over a stove every night after work. Although I knew if I wanted to remain "sick-free", I had to make this a permanent lifestyle change; with my hectic schedule, I had to find quick and easy ways to make it work effectively.

Food for Thought

While blending is a great method to quickly ingest a large amount of vegetables, it is not recommended as a meal replacement or as the only source for any form of food. Juicing and blending have become a popular method to obtain nutrients and protein. While it is a viable option, it is not the best option. It's important to chew your food; the body requires the enzymes created during chewing to digest the food and it signals the brain that you are eating in order to feel full.

Here are some simple tips to healthier eating:

- Instead of canned products, use fresh, frozen, or dry peas or beans. Dry beans are simple to prepare. Pre-soak for 6-8 hours. This can be done before you go to work or bed. Place them in a slow cooker for a few hours, allow to cool off when done, put into zip lock bags and freeze. They are ready to use whenever you need it.
- Cut up fruit and vegetables immediately after purchase. Buy only what you need for that week. Keep them in serving portions in the fridge. It will be ready to eat or cook whenever you need it. This prevents food from sitting too long, rotting, and eventually being tossed out. When you plan your meals, you eat foods that are more nutritious and save money in the process.
- Buy a high-quality blender and blend fresh fruit and vegetable drinks rather than juicing. While juicing may be a healthier option for some, be mindful that the healthy fibers are removed while juicing, making it incomplete in nutrients versus blending the whole item. It's also important to consume cooked food in conjunction with blending. Blending makes it easier to get your daily intake of complete nutrients on the run. Be cautious with blending if you have any sort of fiber intolerance. It is important to alter recipes or information given here to accommodate your particular health issues, lifestyle, taste buds or dietary concerns.
- Do not bring junk or unhealthy food into the house; avoid those aisles at the stores. How likely is it if you are having a

craving that you will get dressed, leave the house and drive to the store to buy it? For most people, when you have the item in the house, it becomes convenient and makes it difficult to exercise willpower not to eat it.
- Make an intentional effort to start preparing at least 2-3 home cook meals a week. More on meal planning in Chapter 9.
- When you do have a treat, buy a small amount and put limitations on how much you eat and what you eat.

SHOCKING FACT: Today, poor food choices, toxic food ingredients, nutritional deficiencies, and lack of physical exercise cause more than 95% of all chronic disease. Family time and family dinnertime are becoming extinct. These behaviors are not just tradition; children who have regular meals with their parent(s) do better in many measures, from better grades, to healthier relationships, to staying out of trouble, and better communication skills. They are 42% less likely to drink alcohol, 50% less likely to smoke cigarettes, and 66% less likely to smoke marijuana. Regular family dinners can protect girls from bulimia, anorexia, and diet pills and has been shown to reduce the incidence of childhood obesity. A study of household routines and obesity on U.S. preschool-aged children, found that kids as young as four years old have a lower risk of obesity if they eat regular family dinners, get sufficient sleep, and don't watch TV on weekdays. Children between the ages of 1-18 are the first generation in two centuries to have a life expectancy shorter than their parents. It is time we make a change.

CHAPTER 9

Secret Three: Eat to Lose - The Power of Food

Healthy Meals on a Dime - Weekly Planned Meals

"If you fail to plan, you plan to fail." - Benjamin Franklin

John and I share the responsibility of cooking every day; initially, it was challenging for the both of us. It was stressful to come home after work and figure out what everyone wanted to eat - only to find out that we did not have the ingredients and needed to make a grocery run. It was also a challenge figuring out something to prepare that would be easy, yet wholesomely nutritious. As John's schedule became more demanding, he cooked less and less. That meant more cooking for me; this was something I dreaded going through almost every day despite the health benefits.

Once again, it became common for us to eat out at least once a week and/or make a stop at the grocery store to get the easy food, boxed, canned or frozen. Although I knew better, I also gave in to convenience to maintain my sanity and reduce stress. This went on for a year, and I started to see fluctuations not just with me, but my family's health. John eventually gave in to eating more processed food because neither of us had the time to cook "real" food. He started to feel the effects of eating unhealthy, he was exhausted throughout the day and many days did not have enough energy to workout. This is not the man that worked out six days a week, including recreational activities, and normally had abundance of energy.

I planned to attend a weeklong conference out-of-state. Immediately, I thought there was no way I could put him through cooking every night, as his job was stressful and he worked many late nights. One of my solutions was to talk my mother into coming over to cook or bring daily meals to the house. She refused and instead suggesting, "Why don't you cook about four or five large meals and store them in the refrigerator?" I thought the idea was brilliant, but not probable. I said, "Do you know how long that will take me?" That seemed to be an impossible task but I attempted it; I did not want my family to starve.

The Challenges of Everyday Cooking

Since that seemed to be the only solution to prevent my family's starvation or eating unhealthy food, I set out to prepare 4-5 meals the day before I left for the conference. I went to the grocery store, without a list, mistake number one. I shopped for the basics; poultry, seafood, vegetables, legumes, beans, and fruits. I returned home and searched online recipes, cookbooks and took recommendations from my family on what they would like to eat, mistake number two. Several hours later, and after a few additional runs to the grocery store to pick up additional items, it was time to prepare and cook. That afternoon I prepared five meals and made a sufficient amount to have both lunch and dinner from each meal. I cut up fruits and vegetables and bagged them for snacks.

I made some extra sandwiches, and baked banana nut muffins and cupcakes for a treat. I felt as if I was Martha Stewart in the kitchen, all the pots were in use, food everywhere and all stove eyelets lit. I was beyond exhausted after spending almost seven hours in the kitchen, not including the time spent grocery shopping. It was a full day's work. I expected it would be time consuming, but not take the entire day. I was overwhelmed and frustrated; my feet, back, and neck hurt to no end by the time I finished. I could not imagine being a chef and cooking a large quantity of meals every day. My mother's brilliant idea did not seem so brilliant anymore. It was very difficult, exhausting, and time-consuming, but I accomplished the mission and I vowed *never* do it again.

Surprising Rave Reviews

When I returned home at the end of the week, John greeted me with flowers at the airport. He could not thank me enough for making such wonderful meals and sparing him the hassle and burden of making breakfast, lunch and dinner every night. He was very appreciative. He said, "I felt more relaxed when I came home from work, knowing that I didn't have to cook or see you aggravated and running around to prepare something." He shared that not having to cook nightly allowed him time to spend with the kids doing something other than just homework during the week; they played board games, went to the park, and watched movies.

The kids enjoyed being able to come home and eat without having to wait hours for someone to get home before they could have a healthy snack or dinner. They enjoyed having the banana nut muffins and cupcakes instead of store bought cookies, granola bars or some other processed snack. My family said they looked forward to coming home, as they anticipated eating their favorite meal. The positive feedback was surprising to hear. I thought they wanted to show appreciation, because they knew the aggravation and frustration that I'd gone through. They continued to make random comments about the positive experience in the following weeks - even though they did not dare ask me to replicate it. However, after several weeks, I decided I wanted to experience what they were describing. I broke my vow and ventured into the kitchen again.

Time to Plan

John and I agreed I would prepare no more than four meals that week, enough to cover lunch and dinner with each for Monday-Thursday. This time I was aware of some of the challenges to expect and how to better plan. I took recommendations from the family, looked up recipes, and made certain that most of the meals required similar ingredients, to cut down on the grocery cost. I prepared a shopping list, and then went to the grocery store. In addition to the four meals, I made one treat, homemade granola bars, and cut up fruits and vegetables that I used for snack packs. Planning made the chore much easier, but it was still time-consuming and exhausting. Although I spent about five hours in the kitchen, it was less than the initial seven hours, and I only made one trip to the grocery store, instead of three as before. Most of all, I looked forward to having time to relax and enjoy some down time during the week as John and the kids did while I was out of town.

Heavenly

That week I felt as if I had died and gone to Heaven. I cannot articulate the stress relief and the weight I felt lifted off my shoulders. I had never felt more at ease and relaxed during a weekday, despite the hectic workday and coming home to family dilemmas. I had the same phenomenon that my family had experienced weeks before. Even morning time was not so chaotic and hectic. There was no yelling, "What am I taking to school or work for lunch?" No fussing, "I don't like that or I don't want that." We were not leaving the house in a mad rush; we packed lunches the night before and it was all a matter of grab and go. John and I did not eat out for lunch that week nor did we grab quick snacks from the vending machines during the day. In the evening, I came home from work or from running the children around to extracurricular activities without having to stand in a line at the grocery store or some fast food place.

I looked forward to going home. I felt more relaxed and interacted more with my family instead of standing over a hot stove for an hour or more. We ate as a family, completed schoolwork and had enough time for a movie or other family activities on most nights – and that literally never happened during the week, unless of course we had take-out. It was truly an amazing feeling. I no longer felt stressed about rushing home and preparing a meal. I had more time to spend with my family, and was also more patient when assisting with homework without being exhausted by the end of the night. The family also enjoyed not having a huge kitchen clean up every evening; instead, we were able to spend that time more productively, and we all loved it.

As time passed I purchased cookbooks, and by this time the Internet was easily accessible so I downloaded recipes. I had a mindset shift about the cooking - I did not perceive cooking as a negative and grueling activity anymore. I started to enjoy pre-planning and cooking because of all the benefits; eating healthier meals, improving our health, less stress, and more family time during the week. I loved seeing my family's face of delight, enjoying meals I had naturally prepared and as a result, my confidence in the kitchen was heightened. I began receiving compliments from my family and friends about my meals, especially my spinach and mushroom lasagna (see Recipes section). As my confidence increased, I made meals that were more elaborate and ventured out with exotic recipes. I cooked on my off days; therefore, I had more time to experiment with ingredients and recipes. I was not in a rush to prepare a meal as I did during the week just to satisfy hungry bellies.

I typically made at least two simple meals and two elaborate meals, yet it did not increase my time in the kitchen. The elaborate meals included Jambalaya, Crab Cakes, Stuffed Salmon, Gumbo, Chicken Curry, or Stewed Oxtail. John agreed he and the kids would cook Friday through Sunday, or would eat any leftovers from the week. My family loved the fact that I was becoming a "chef" and they did not have to eat the same boring meals week after week.

Whenever I experimented with a new dish for the first time, I made it according to the recipe; the next time I made changes according to my family's taste buds. In addition, if we did not like a new recipe, I knew not to make it again. Seeing the smiles on their faces each week was incentive enough for me to continue, week after week, month after month, and year after year. My family and I are now so accustomed to home-cooked meals; we dislike eating out because it usually costs too much and very rarely is the food better than mine, not to toot my own horn. This is from the same person who could not boil an egg.

Price vs. Cost

I loved the perks of planning and preparing meals. The cost of being less stressed, enjoying time with the family, being less exhausted, saving money and achieving wellness far outweighed the price I paid by giving up several hours on a Saturday or Sunday preparing our meals. Oftentimes, we did not have to cook on the weekend or eat out since there were enough leftovers from the weekly meals. The greatest surprise came when I noticed that I was not going over my food budget each week and less food was wasted. Weekly meal planning cut my food budget by 30%. I cooked whatever I purchased that week and there was rarely any waste. The prepared food was stored in containers and kept in the fridge or freezer. The majority of people I talk to think they cannot eat healthy on a budget, but I am here to tell you yes you can. When you think of the cost per meal you prepared versus a fast food meal, on average, it's an enormous savings.

Weekly meal planning turned into a regular family event. We typically cooked on Sunday after church, or Saturday if the kids did not have any extracurricular events. Initially, I did it alone, but later I encouraged the family to assist. They chopped, sliced, or diced, seasoned, and did anything to help the process move along faster; they knew as long as I was in the kitchen, we did not leave the house. Within 90 days, I was preparing 4-5 meals in less than four hours.

Previously, I averaged 1-1 ½ hours a day for each meal - so comparatively, 4 hours in one day preparing 4-5 meals plus snacks was a walk in the park. Overall, I saved 2-4 hours a week than if I cooked a meal every day. *Hallelujah!* I finally felt as if we were on the right track as a family, moving towards living healthier lifestyles. Planning weekly meals made a huge impact on our overall wellness and savings.

"Instead of going out to dinner, buy good food. Cooking at home shows such affection. In a bad economy, it's more important to make yourself feel good." - Ina Garten

The extra time we had during the week allowed for more family interaction; we designated Wednesdays as family game night. Most Friday nights we made nachos or tacos with ground turkey, or homemade chicken and seafood pizza (see Recipes section); afterwards we did something fun outside the house. Once every other month on Friday night, we had a takeout pizza, - cheese-less, chicken and vegetables for John (he refused to eat dairy, see Chapter 11), and the kids and I ate cheese and pepperoni, that was our "treat" food. Over the next several months, we were eating less fast and processed food, and generally leading a healthier and more relaxed lifestyle. It looked as if only sunny skies were ahead. After about six months, my health concerns were consistently under control and I did not need to check my blood sugar daily. I'd normally refill my purse with glucose tablets weekly, but I hadn't done that in several months.

I loved the benefits of pre-planning weekly meals so much that I am still doing it nine years later and even now as an empty nester. It has become such a habit and not a burden - even on vacation, we usually stay in places with a kitchen and take a couple hours the first day to make our meals and snacks. We plan the meals before leaving home and pack small amounts of spices and condiments into zip lock bags, to avoid the extra cost. Let's hear it for saving money and still eating healthy while on vacation! John is a finance guru, and according to his calculations, pre-planning and cooking vacation meals cuts the vacation food cost by more than 70%. Hence, you can also vacation on a budget.

Just recently, while on vacation, John and I treated ourselves to a meal at a local sushi restaurant. We managed to walk away with a reasonable tab of $68 before gratuity. We thought it was well worth it since we enjoyed the food and it's one of our favorite places in Phoenix. That feeling quickly wore off after leaving the grocery store. We purchased food for the week to prepare our meals as we usually do while out of town. The bill came of $64. We spent more money for one meal than we did for groceries at a local health food store for a week. Wow! Although eating out is acceptable while living a healthy lifestyle, doing so excessively can break your budget as well as contribute to health issues.

Practical tips to start weekly planned meals:

1. Plan and cook 3-4 weekly simple meals on your day off. Get the family's input about what they would like to eat that week; remember you can't please everyone. Find meals with similar basic ingredients. Doing so will prevent buying lots of food, condiments and spices you don't use very often.

2. If there's a recipe that calls for a particular spice you would not normally use, go to a health food store and buy only the amount you need from the bulk section. For example, a recipe calls for 2 teaspoons (.33 oz.) pumpkin spice - instead of buying a one ounce jar at the average price of $5 that you won't use in the near future, buy .33 ounce for less than $.50 cents from bulk.

3. Plan at least 1-2 treats and 3-4 various snacks. This could include fruit and vegetables. Cut them up and individually pack them.

4. Make a list of ingredients needed and take it to the grocery store. Stick to the meats and produce section to avoid buying unnecessary and processed items.

5. Start by prepping your food; cut up vegetables and season meats before you actually start to cook. Some items may require marinating; do those first.

6. Once the food is cooked and cooled, separate into serving sizes, refrigerate or freeze for later use.

7. It's a good idea to label your food containers with a dry erase pen or paper labels so you know how long it's been stored and can quickly identify it in the freezer. Note: The dry erase easily comes off with vinegar or rubbing alcohol.

8. Take note, if you have never experienced this phenomenon, try it out for 90 days and experience less stress, more family time, gain better health, save money, lose weight, and increase your energy.

9. Check in on how your family feels about working together in the kitchen to create a level of harmony and good health that is best achieved when food is prepared in a loving manner, and eaten slowly with others. There are no more excuses about time and schedules for unhealthy eating. Instead, let us look at why preparing food is a win-win situation for everyone. During the week, relax and enjoy some "me time" or time with your family! Post your feedback on www.facebook.com/parkerlifestyle.

SHOCKING FACT: A poll taken by "Real Money" showed that 2 out of 3 people believed they were spending too much money on home cooked meals and food. They did a challenge of a husband going to a restaurant, ordering a whole chicken, rice, and beans dinner and the wife cooked fish and vegetables at home. He clocked in at 31 minutes and she at 22 minutes to complete the task, at a cost $22 for the restaurant meal and $12 for the home-cooked meal for two people. In addition to living a healthier lifestyle, and all the other perks discussed, you save time and money when you cook at home.

CHAPTER 10

It's Never Too Late: EAT this, NOT this

"Excellence is an art won by training and habituation. We do not act rightly because we have virtue or excellence, but we rather have those because we have acted rightly. We are what we repeatedly do. Excellence, then, is not an act, but a habit." - Aristotle

Creatures of Habit

I wanted to live a longer life, a life free from worrying about passing out at the wheel and endangering my family, others, or myself - a life free from medication and the harmful effects of diabetes and other health concerns. I wanted to live a healthier lifestyle, and since I loved to eat, I had to figure out how to do so without putting my health in danger. I wanted to feel on the inside what everyone saw on the outside. Making "healthier" choices was a huge part of that change. I realized it was realistic to live without getting headaches, feeling nauseous, passing out, shakiness, and poking myself daily to check my sugar levels. Developing new eating habits and effectively changing my mindset about what I wanted my life to look like would be a good start to achieve this goal. I accepted that several factors, including eating and recreational habits, needed to change in order for my health to change. When I made changes with my lifestyle, I not only changed the destiny of my life, but my family's life and that of future generations.

Do Not Judge a Book by its Cover

"You are so beautiful and look healthy," a compliment I often received, but little did they know I was not always so healthy on the inside. I accepted that I did not know what I did not know. No one, including healthcare professionals, educated me about diabetes, the potential danger in the food I was eating, or the impact of not managing life stressors. As difficult and uncomfortable as it was to get out of my unhealthy comfort zone, I realized I had to make *permanent* changes; it was a matter of life or death.

Developing healthier habits meant an overall lifestyle change, not a 21-day challenge or a diet. It required a new comfort zone and permanent way of thinking about my life. A lifestyle change does not entail drastic overnight changes, eating foods you do not enjoy, or changing everything in your pantry. It does mean eating more passionately with awareness of ingredients in food and being intentional about choices. These subtle changes will make a huge impact that can result in a total transformation from the inside and out.

Feeling Energized

During my initial transition, I was not aware of the potential dangers in the foods that I thought were quick, easy, and inexpensive. It was not until the last few years that more information became readily available, which better explained the effects of these ingredients on our health (see Chapter 6). Products such as ketchup, canned tomatoes, or frozen meals should be relatively "healthy" food; it's how it is processed that renders it an unhealthy option.

Avoiding and limiting "processed foods" was the beginning of my solution to defy diabetes and other health concerns naturally. Once I began changing how and what I ate, I noticed that my sugar levels became more stable over time. I also noticed I had more energy and no longer felt tired by midday. I was not completely exhausted and napping as soon as I arrived home from work. The 30 extra pounds I gained over the years, which I thought was normal and a result of aging, began to melt away. These were a few of the positive results I had after I eliminated most processed food from my life; I also reduced my stress level and practiced better sleep habits. I did not understand the correlation with the central nervous system and food, and my healthcare professionals did not explain this to me. At the time, I identified bits and pieces of information, but nothing to the degree of what I am sharing with you. Most of this I discovered as I evolved and explored, but there are now many studies to confirm that eating habits play a significant role in our overall wellness. I continued to be disciplined and practiced incremental changes throughout the years, witnessing my transformation and creating a lifestyle change.

It's Never Too Late

If you already have health concerns...arthritis, high blood pressure, hormonal issues etc., it's not too late to make a change. Make a decision to change your lifestyle today using the methods discussed here. Most of the foods we eat are "useless" food sources, a waste of money, and a potential cause of many health risks. Begin to think outside of the cereal box.

Here are some suggestions for alternative ingredients:

EAT This	**NOT This**
Wild rice	White rice or flour
Rooibos, herbal, green/white tea	Coffee or energy drinks
Water with lemon or lime	Soda or fruit drinks
Dark-colored fruits	Dried fruits
Coconut nectar or stevia	Artificial sweeteners
Almond or cashew butter	Peanut butter
Nut or plant based products	Dairy products and Soy
Fish, chicken, turkey	Red meat
Grass fed butter	Margarine
Dark chocolate 70% or higher	Milk or white chocolate
Sweet or red potatoes	White potatoes
Fresh or frozen vegetables	Canned vegetables
Olive oil with lemon	Salad dressing
Sprouted bread	White or wheat bread
Pink Himalayan Sea Salt	Iodized table salt

SHOCKING FACT: There are added ingredients such as sodium, sugars, dairy, hydrogenated oils, and artificial preservatives and colors in processed foods, many of which are listed under various names. Current research shows these ingredients have little nutritional value and many empty calories. In addition, the added ingredients can cause inflammation, insulin and blood sugar instability, and other health concerns. Increased hyperactivity and Attention Deficit Hyperactivity Disorder (ADHD) have been linked to artificial color such as yellow 5, blue 1, and red 40. Reports have revealed chemical traces of aluminum and BPA in most canned products; research has shown that aluminum is possibly one of the contributing factors to Alzheimer while BPA may be a contributing factor to certain cancers.

CHAPTER 11

Got Milk?!?

"But, the real secret to long-life good health is actually the opposite: Let your body take care of you." - Deepak Chopra.

Why Dairy Is NOT Your Friend?

There is a common argument against consuming animal milk products and many health risks attributed to its consumption. Why is it that this "natural" product is unnatural for humans to consume? The evolutionary perspective is that a mother's milk, animal or human, is needed to provide nutrients to the baby for growth and development. Before the increase in human population and evolution of commercialized agriculture, humans drank their mother's milk as infants only.

Despite popular demand, research has shown that consuming dairy products does not do the body good. There seems to be more disadvantages than advantages to ingesting this staple product. There are reasons why many of us are lactose intolerant - we lack the enzyme, lactase, which helps to digest animal-based dairy products. This can contribute to conditions such as digestive issues, hormonal imbalance, osteoporosis, and risk of cancer. It carries high toxins that can weaken the immune system, and disrupt the reproductive and central nervous systems. It can also trigger skin conditions, sinus problems, inflammation, ear infections, and can lead to an increased risk of Parkinson's disease in men.

Sinus infections and colds began to plague my daughter again as she entered her teenage years, at times coughing up huge chunks of bacteria balls and mucus, known as tonsil stones. Doctors said they did not know what was causing these problems and suggested removing her tonsils. Similar symptoms began to emerge with John, including a dry cough. Both he and my daughter described a feeling that "something was stuck in their throat." This became progressively worse over a two-year period. We finally went to an Ear, Nose and Throat Specialist, who said, "It's not a major problem, just a buildup of mucus and there is nothing to do about that, but when the problem arises take an antibiotic." At that point, we had invested so much into changing our health and lifestyle, we had no idea why they had this mucus build up, but we knew we had to re-evaluate our food consumption. Education has taught us that nothing is happening to the body that we are not causing in some manner.

I began studying and researching mucus, the culprit. We discovered that what the doctors referred to as "not a problem, just mucus" could in fact be symptoms related to the use of dairy products. Researchers referred to the buildup of mucus as Phlegm. Studies I reviewed consistently showed a correlation between dairy products and increased inflammation due to mucus or phlegm in the body. An article published by Harvard Health states that *inflammation* is one of the main causes of sinus problems, digestive issues, arthritis, heart disease, stroke, kidney disease, cancer and diabetes. This information provided guidance as to why me and my family were having digestive issues, constipation, aching joints, sinus infection, and tonsil stones. Concerns that were stated to be normal were actually abnormal and could have been avoided by what we were ingesting.

What is Phlegm and do you have it?

According to the definition in the medical dictionary, phlegm is an inflammation, a fluid or semifluid substance also referred to as humor, caused by heat. It is a liquid secreted by the mucous membranes of mammals. Its definition is limited to the mucus produced by the respiratory system (it excludes the nasal passages), and particularly, which is expelled by coughing (sputum).

Mucus is something we all have in our system as it plays an active role in keeping our bodies healthy. Its main job is to protect the body from irritants like bacteria, viruses or allergens. When it becomes out of balance or we have too much in our system, that is when it creates a health risk. As with most things within our body, we have to create a happy balance. Dr. Noel Rose, the director of auto-immunology at Johns Hopkins, declares, "The cause of autoimmune disease is multifactorial. Due to the significant increase of toxins over the last few decades, the body is in overload and is having difficulty recognizing between self and non-self." This causes it to be out of balance and creates many of the health epidemics we are seeing today.

Time to Experiment

How often have you heard the slogan, "Milk does the body good." Most Western healthcare professionals encourage its consumption for calcium and vitamin D nutrients. They also profess it as a great source for protein and probiotic cultures needed for great health. Yet, other research shows that milk is not the optimal choice to obtain these nutrients. Dairy intake could have attributed to my family's health problems and we needed to make a change. We decided to experiment and began the process of removing it completely from our diet. We took all dairy products out of our household for a month. We had no choice, we went cold turkey, considering we all were having problems related to dairy. I was lactose intolerant, took Lactaid tablets, digestive enzymes and drank lactose-free milk to alleviate the symptoms. This was the perfect reason for me to stop and observe the effects.

In addition, I knew from experience that waiting for a drastic symptom to occur before I took action, was not the best option. Even though I did not have obvious symptoms as my family, it was causing problems in my body unbeknownst to me. Although we had been diligent with changing many of our dietary habits, dairy was more difficult to give up. We bought into what healthcare professionals were calling benefits for using dairy. I think I was in denial or just did not want to accept the fact that this "natural" product could potentially be harmful. John had stopped eating cheese years prior, but occasionally used some other dairy products such as 2% milk and sour cream. Yet, his body had an imbalance of mucus. Considering we did not want to use any other alternative for milk, we stopped eating the "sugary" cereal and the occasional pizza. Ultimately, the transition worked out great; we not only stopped dairy, but also decreased the undesirable sugary cereals. We will discuss later why most cereal and pizza should be avoided.

Charles de Gaulle said, *"How can you govern a country which has 246 varieties of cheese?"*

Giving up milk and cheese was a difficult change for my daughter and me. John could go cold turkey on almost anything he sets his mind to. We have different personalities; therefore, a weaning process was best to ensure my success. One day, I discovered a documentary where they asked a thought-provoking question, "Why are humans the only species who drink another animal's milk well into adulthood?" Actually, most, if not all baby animals drink milk from their mother. It all started to make sense to me. Our bodies will accept animal or synthetic milk only at the infancy development stage. Studies found that continuing to drink milk into adulthood could result in an increase of phlegm, tonsil stones or inflammation. The body deems it a foreign object due to the chemicals used during processing. Many of you may not always respond with visible health concerns as with my family, but there is enough evidence to prove that the risk of consuming some dairy products is greater than the reward.

Changing our attitude and behaviors toward dairy products was a gradual change. Initially, we went from whole milk to 2% milk. After discovering, they use more sugar and chemicals to render milk anything less than "whole", we switched back to whole milk. To decrease the use of milk and cereal each morning, we used a plant-based protein to make fruit smoothies, eggs on sprouted bread, or oatmeal. At the time, we did not have many of the substitutes or alternatives for milk readily available that are now popular, i.e., coconut, rice, almond, hemp or hazelnut milk. Although soymilk was available, we could not stomach the taste. Many years later, researchers are still debating if soy is responsible for hormonal problems and possibly certain types of cancer. I finally followed my husband and went cold turkey. Now, I can say that my family is about 98% dairy-free. Most importantly, I avoid bringing it into the house, which made it easier to avoid consumption and temptation.

Within several months of giving up the dairy, John's cough and the tonsil stones that had previously clogged his throat were gone. My daughter no longer dealt with sinus headache, cold, or ear infections on a weekly basis. At that point, we knew we had to stick to the drastic changes we had made and I did not have to fight with my daughter anymore to convince her why we should avoid dairy products. The results spoke for themselves, and since she did not like being in pain and constantly sick, she did not dispute it. Although I originally thought I did not have a reaction to dairy, except for digestive issues, I was wrong. The pain and stiffness in my joints dissipated shortly after discontinuing its use. Healthcare professionals said the joint pain was due to arthritis and aging. Normally we do not correlate pain, allergies, or indications like lactose intolerance as symptoms related to what we are eating; however, more often than you may think, there is a correlation.

Food for thought

Arthritis is typically a result of chronic inflammation in your body. Anything *-itis* means chronic inflammation. Inflammation is the body's attempt at self-protection to remove harmful stimuli and begin the healing process. Inflammation becomes chronic when the body's mucus is out of balance. As a result, the immune system begins to attack healthy tissue, causing enormous pain. Chronic inflammation can eventually cause several conditions, including some cancers, rheumatoid arthritis, atherosclerosis, periodontitis and hay fever.

Is Dairy for you?

Most people who have some sensitivity to gluten generally have issues with dairy, including raw dairy. However, most people do not realize they have sensitivity because it may be subtle, or we may not attribute it to something we are ingesting. The sensitivity to it does not always manifest itself in the typical gassy/bloating ways. In my family's case, the healthcare provider diagnosed the problem of excessive mucus and chronic inflammation, but did not recommend a permanent solution nor did they explain why this occurred. Inflammation symptoms can manifest in a variety of ways such as sinus problems, ear infections, low energy, fogginess, and joint pain. Stomach pains, bloating, diarrhea, gas, and constipation are often mistaken as Irritable Bowel Syndrome (IBS). Other symptoms include acne or rash breakouts, regular yeast infections, autoimmune issues, and dry or itchy skin. Is it a coincidence or substantiated evidence that since avoiding dairy, my family has not experienced any of those aforementioned problems? Being the "researcher" that he is, John experimented periodically with milk to confirm whether it triggered the same problems as before - and time after time, the symptoms returned.

When I first started this journey over seven years ago, there were not as many alternatives readily available for non-dairy products nor was there as much research as there is today. Now, there are many tasty non-dairy, no-soy alternatives on the market to make this lifestyle change a smooth transition.

Try these alternatives:

- Cheese alternative: Daiya products. To my knowledge, it does not contain any soy products and it melts easily, so you can still enjoy a good grilled cheese sandwich. It comes in cheddar, Swiss, provolone, and mozzarella.
- Almond, rice, or coconut milk instead of whole milk, 2%, skim milk or soymilk.
- Coconut yogurt instead of Greek yogurt.
- Instead of sugary cereals with milk, use plant or nut based milk with oatmeal (not instant). Add a portion of non-dairy protein or make a non-dairy based protein smoothie, using one serving of fruit.
- Other alternatives include eggs on rye/whole grain/sprouted bread; an apple with peanut or almond butter; fruit and nuts in almond milk. Be creative, there is a world of healthier and flavorful alternatives.

Many people have been led to believe that the only way you can get sufficient protein and calcium is with dairy products - which is a myth. Many plants, vegetables, fish, beans, and legumes provide the daily allowance of calcium and protein. Breakfast does not always have to be the traditional "All American Breakfast" (cereal, pancakes, bacon or eggs). My favorite breakfast foods are a 15 bean or lentil soup; walnuts, almonds and pine nuts mixed with berries and almond milk. Both provide adequate fiber, protein, calcium, and other daily-required nutrients.

SHOCKING FACT: What we eat may not only cause a buildup of inflammation in the body, but it can set the stage for other problems such as obesity, heart disease and diabetes. Here is a list of foods known to trigger chronic inflammation: Sugar, Saturated Fats, Trans

Fat, Omega 6 Fatty Acids, Refined Carbohydrates, MSG, Gluten, Casein, Aspartame, and Alcohol. It does not mean you cannot eat any of these ingredients; it just means to limit usage.

CHAPTER 12

The Skinny on Carbs

"Not all carbs are created equal." - Unknown

Don't Believe the Hype

Contrary to popular belief, carbohydrates are not all created equal. The better news is that not all carbs are bad. Based on the chemical composition and how the body processes carbohydrates is what makes it simple, yet complex. The problem with carbohydrates is not the carbohydrates themselves, but the confusion on what is good and what is not. It is no wonder we get frustrated and eat whatever because we are overloaded and puzzled with information, and do not know what to believe. I hope that I can help set the record straight. I have had to do in-depth research, because it seems everything I love to eat includes carbs. All the hype says to stay clear of it, yet my body was telling me differently when I did not have them.

Sometimes we may load up on cookies, pastries, bread, donuts, potato chips, and cakes because we enjoy them and they give us a burst of energy. These are *simple carbohydrates*, and that means it is high in sugar and other processed items. It gives you a burst of energy, but it does not last very long. Before we go further, let me explain Simple versus Complex Carbohydrates.

Carbohydrates become simple or "bad carbs," when the ingredients are refined and stripped of its nutrients. Examples include instant oatmeal, most breakfast cereal, dinner rolls, cookies, or pastries to name a few. Most simple carbohydrates are easily digested due to its basic ingredients such as sugars or sugar substitutes. These sugars go directly into the bloodstream, giving you that jolt of energy, causing spikes in blood sugar levels (see Chapter 2). The higher a product is in sugar content and lower in fiber, the worse it is and the more harmful the effects on the body and organs.

Carbohydrates, in and of themselves, are *not* bad. *Complex carbohydrates*, "good carbs," are something our body needs in order to fuel our system. Complex carbohydrates have the components of sugar, starch and fiber. They include items such as whole grains, legumes, nuts, beans, sweet potatoes, and other root vegetables. Some simple carbohydrates, such as fruits and vegetables are exception to the rule because they act like complex carbs in the body. Complex carbs form a longer chain of sugar molecules; therefore, it takes longer to digest, and *does not* cause a sudden spike in blood sugar. They help us feel full for a longer period. In consuming them, we typically will not overeat and feel hungry, making them vital components in healthier eating and weight loss.

Although complex carbohydrates provide the body energy and are needed to maintain good health, we must be cautious of how much we consume according to body weight and activity levels. There are many controversies surrounding carbs and many trends have come and gone. More studies than not have shown that complex carbs "does the body good." For example, carbohydrate loading is a technique originally devised in the mid-1900s for high-endurance and high-activity level athletes to increase their muscle's glycogen storage level. It is believed that we may be able to exercise longer before fatigue sets in when we undergo carbohydrate loading. Trained athletes with professional guidance usually participate in carbohydrate loading; it is not something I would suggest you do as a non-athlete or without professional assistance. It is important to know that complex carbohydrates are a vital component to every meal. Complex carbohydrates provide us with an even amount of energy without the blood sugar spikes that are common with simple carbs.

There are some basic principles to help you achieve the appropriate portion of daily carbohydrates. The amount of carb intake depends on age, gender, body composition, activity levels, personal preference and current metabolic levels. The Health Science Academy suggests a carb intake of 3-5 grams per kilogram of body weight, depending on physical activity level. This means for most of us, roughly 30-35% of your daily calorie requirements should come from natural protein, 10-15% from essential fats, and the remaining 50-60% from complex carbohydrates. If you simply remove the "bad" carbs from your diet, then you will be well on your way to better health. Even though there is no foolproof scientific explanation of how much carbs each individual requires, research shows the following guidelines to be effective:

100-150 Grams per Day - This amount is a moderate intake appropriate for people who are lean and have an active lifestyle. It is possible to lose weight at this level but it may require you to count calories. At this level, you can eat all the vegetables you want, 1-2 servings of fruit/day and some starchy items like sweet potato and healthier grains, beans and legumes.

50-100 Grams per Day - This level is great if you want to lose weight effortlessly. It's important to allow a bit of complex carbs for energy. Practice the same as above with less starchy food intake.

20-50 Grams per Day - This is the ideal level for those who really want to lose weight fast or have diabetes. Beware, low carbs does not mean no-carbs; eat less starchy food.

We are all unique and we each have different requirements. What works for one person may not work for you. Experiment!

What do your cravings mean?

Not all simple carbs are created equal. Fruits and vegetables are actually simple carbohydrates. The body processes it as complex carbs because of the high fiber content. The fiber in fruits and vegetables determines the digestion rate of how the body processes its sugar content. They slow down the digestion process, making them a bit more like complex carbohydrates. In addition, avoid complex carbs like white potatoes and white rice due to how it's process in the body - it's similar to simple carbs - these are composed of basic sugars although they appear drastically different from other foods in the category, i.e. cookies and cakes, which are processed or fake foods.

Generally, we eat certain foods out of habit or we crave a particular food because the body is lacking nutrients. Find healthy alternatives for your cravings. If you are craving potato chips, your body may be craving the carb due to low serotonin levels, happy chemical, or you may be dehydrated and the body wants the salt/sodium. Instead of potato chips, eat kale chips, celery or toasted edamame. Make certain to combine the carbs with some Omega 3 fatty acid and protein to include Anchovies, Bluefish, Herring, Mackerel, Salmon (wild fish has more omega-3s than farmed), Sardines, and Tuna, for the most efficient nutrient absorption. See Chapter 17 for more nutritional facts and benefits of Omega 3.

Similar to potato chip cravings, night time sweet cravings usually mean the body either did not get enough nutrients or had too much sugar throughout the day. Therefore, the body is struggling to maintain its energy levels, and insulin levels are not stable. I eat meals/snacks higher in protein and fiber when I crave carbs or sweets at night. To satisfy my late night sweet craving my favorite snack is PB&J; using one-tablespoon almond butter and half-teaspoon natural fruit preserves on one slice of sprouted bread. Another favorite, 4 - 6 prunes with one tablespoon of almond butter. Keep in mind prunes, although high in fiber, are also high in sugar as with most dried fruits. Be mindful of your daily sugar intake; if it is high during the day, a prune snack may not be the best option for you. We can extinguish cravings when we give the body what it needs during the day. When you do have cravings, you don't have to eat the "bad stuff." Later, I will share some recipes for treats and alternative options to cupcakes, brownies, and popsicles that are healthier than store bought items. The basic rule of thumb: avoid the processed food and eat in moderation.

Your Back Fat Is Showing

One day while on my third date with John, I got up from the sofa to grab us some water. While walking away from him, I discretely pulled at my shirt to cover my mid-section - about, which he remarked, "Your back fat is showing." I knew deep down he meant no harm and that it was just his sick sense of humor. Nonetheless, I was very upset and offended by this comment. I could not believe he said that to me - either he felt too comfortable after only three dates, or he was that inconsiderate and insensitive. I thought, "You can get the heck out," and wanted to say a few other things to him.

It was unlike me to hold my tongue but I did; I thought he would plead temporary insanity. I kept calm and thought, "Okay, this is the last date for you, mister, I got the perfect body." I had been gaining a few pounds, but I thought it was due to age or hormonal changes, and it was normal. Yet, I was very conscientious and sensitive about my mid-section in particulate. I thought I was doing really well with my health concerns, so I felt very offended by his comment. I had recently started working out again (somewhat) and diligently worked to break "bad" eating habits.

When I returned to the sofa, a blind man could see I was upset - and so did John. He gave me such a sincere and honest apology; I could not help but forgive him. At the time, he was not aware of the demons (hypoglycemia and diabetes) I had been dealing with for the last few years. The amazing thing was that as cynical as the comment was, there was no malice intended, and I forgave him. Initially, I felt intimidated by his healthy lifestyle; he was proud of it, as he should have been. Throughout our conversation, he was humble and willing to help me find solutions to lose the weight. That incident allowed us an opportunity to have a conversation about my weight.

The information he shared pertaining to fitness and health suggested a high level of knowledge. He explained that my growing mid-section could be a sign of health issues and suggested that I continue to improve my eating habits, which was no surprise. What was surprising is when he said I should consider changing up my physical activity level to include more cardio exercise. He suggested decreasing simple carbohydrates, sugar, and increasing protein; he also indicated that other aspects like stress was probably a factor. I explained that I had been avoiding soda, candy, and processed foods, but I ate many carbohydrates. I ate rice, potato, flour, roti (East and West Indian bread made from flour), milk, cheese and crackers, (my 'ole' go-to snack), and bread because I did not think those items were unhealthy. My carb intake was not only high considering my low activity level, but as I explained earlier in this chapter, I ate all of the wrong kinds of carbs, giving my body too much sugar which was not being appropriately used. At that time, I did not know there was a difference in the type of carbohydrates, good versus bad.

Frustration Sets In

After that conversation, I was a little frustrated and wondered what was the point of being healthy if I had to give up all the foods I enjoyed. What else would there be left to eat? I started looking at diets to lose the weight instead of working on being healthy. In hindsight, that was not the best approach. Dieting did not create permanency or long-term effects or habits (see Chapter 3). However, I did not know that at the time and went into action mode to lose the extra inches.

A few weeks after the "back fat" conversation, I saw an infomercial on a popular "no carb" diet. It seemed almost perfect. I was clueless as to what I could eat without starving myself and that diet - high-protein intake and little to no carbohydrates - gave me some guidance. Here was a reputable "diet" from a trained medical doctor, who promoted no carbohydrates; this confirmed John's suggestions and therefore I thought, "It's a sure weight loss plan." At that point, I was still not in the right mindset because my goal should have been about my health rather than losing weight. At the time, my physical appearance was important to me, especially since I had this handsome, athletic, and healthy man in my life; I *had* to look just as good.

Die-At-It (Diet)

I started this new diet or what I like to refer to as "die-at-it." I went cold turkey and eliminated oatmeal, breads, rice, pasta, potatoes, and pretty much anything carbs. It did not take me as long to undergo this change as I did with kicking the soda and candy habit, yet it was still challenging. My thought was after shedding the pounds, I would resume my normal eating habits in moderation and should be able to maintain my weight. Functioning on zero carbohydrates was challenging for me as I was constantly hungry and did not enjoy the recipes they suggested.

This plan did not last long. Within less than two months, my blood sugar level was fluctuating and the hypoglycemic episodes returned, but the inches were coming off. I was completely confused; I didn't quite know how to adjust my eating habits. My options were to eat the carbohydrates and have more energy, or to eat no carbs and lose weight with unstable blood sugar levels and fatigue. What was I to do? It did not make sense and my body went against what I was reading according to this particular diet. I felt lost, confused and frustrated once again. I wanted to hire a personal trainer, but it was not within my budget, and most of them, from previous inquiries, were only versed in exercise and had little expertise in nutrition.

It is amazing how people have come into my life at the right time. I met a personal trainer while attending an event. During our conversation, I shared my struggles and the new diet I had started. She said removing all carbohydrates is one of the worst things anyone could do, particularly if you are active and diabetic. It totally blew me away. She explained everything I was experiencing without me disclosing many details to her - low energy, dizziness, and low blood sugar - she was precise with the information. Finally, I thought, a personal trainer who knew something about nutrition and the effects it can have on the body. I later discovered she was also a certified holistic nutritionist. She encouraged me to take a few nutrition classes to have a better understanding of complex versus simple carbohydrates and the effects they have on the body. She cautioned me, however, that the information taught was from a Western Medicine perspective, and not from alternative medicine. There is a slight variation between the two practices; the information I am sharing is from a Natural Health perspective.

Answer to My Prayer

The personal trainer further explained that most people need to eat carbohydrates, but it should be COMPLEX Carbohydrates and only selected SIMPLE Carbohydrates (fruits and vegetables, not white bread and pasta). To fuel the body we need carbohydrates, but at the time, I did not know there was a difference between simple and complex carbohydrates. Although John knew this information, he did not explain that aspect to me, because he assumed I knew. I learned that complex carbs are the primary fuel for the central nervous system, which cannot fully function without them. No wonder I felt such fatigue; my body was not getting the fuel it needed to perform, especially during my workouts. When insulin levels are chronically too low, which could happen with low carb diets, muscle protein breakdown increases and a lack of protein synthesis occurs.

Carbohydrates help to prime the metabolic system in burning fat. The trainer further explained when the metabolic system adapts to prolonged low-carb/high-fat/high-protein diets, it can cause the system to decrease significantly over time. Therefore, my initial weight loss would have been temporary, and I probably would have gained even more weight if I continued on that particular diet.

Once I was better informed about complex carbohydrates and incorporated the appropriate amounts, it improved my sugar levels, increased my energy, and helped me shed weight. In addition, I incorporated cardiovascular exercises including step aerobics, line dancing and swimming. They were more enjoyable to me than walking or running on a treadmill. The trainer also introduced me to the elliptical machine and StairMaster, which became my favorite means to obtain an intense cardio workout. When weather permitted, I engaged in outdoor activities, running the bleachers at the local high school, hiking and rollerblading at the park. Finally, my health was on the right course and I said goodbye to the pounds. More importantly, I could eat bread (sprouted), potatoes (red), and rice (brown or wild) and did not feel I was giving up the foods I loved.

What is the Glycemic Index?

According to the American Society of Nutrition, the glycemic index is a measurement of sugar and carbohydrate in food and their impact on blood sugar levels. When eating natural sugars and complex carbohydrates, it is important to consider glycemic levels. Glycemic levels are important not just for diabetics, but also for everyone. When speaking of simple carbohydrates, in most cases it refers to high sugars, starch, and empty calories. Contrary to popular opinion, sugar is not the number one enemy, it's the form of sugar and how much we ingest - many health issues are predicated on the amount of simple sugar ingested routinely.

For optimal health, choose foods in the lower Glycemic Index (GI) category, avoid the high category, and go easy on those in between (see the chart below). It will be much easier for American consumers to determine the glycemic levels of a product if manufacturers put a symbol on packaging as they do in Australia. Until then, take control of your health and use information such as what's shared in this book. It is important to have a glycemic index chart close by until you become familiar with certain foods and how it affects you.

Follow the sample chart below or visit glycemicindex.com for more specific information by food item.

- Low Glycemic Index - GI of 55 or less: Most fruits, vegetables, beans, minimally processed whole grains, and nuts.
- Medium Glycemic Index - GI of 56-69: Sweet potatoes, corn, brown rice, couscous, and regular pancakes (one six-inch pancake has a GI of 67).
- High Glycemic Index - GI of 70 and higher: White bread, white rice, white potatoes, cakes, bagels, most cereals, jellybeans, most crackers, cookies, candy, pastries, dried fruit and most packaged breakfast cereals.
- Monitoring your glycemic index levels in food is an effective way to help maintain or lose weight, prevent fatigue, decrease and combat cholesterol, cardiovascular disease, and blood sugar levels.

Choose This:

- *Complex Carbohydrates* - Vegetables, legumes, beans, sprouted grains, rolled or steel oats, and bran.
- Caution: Fruits and root vegetables are considered simple carbs but act as complex carbs in the body. Therefore, use them in moderation.

Not This:

- *Simple Carbohydrates* - White bread, white rice, white potatoes, white pasta, soda, artificial syrups and sugar, pastries, cookies, and most desserts. Before purchasing items such as granola bars, look at the ingredients; if it resembles a candy bar more than oatmeal, then it performs like a simple carbohydrate.

Here are some simple tips to help break the "bad" carb addiction:

- Overall, studies show that complex carbohydrates are needed, along with protein and essential fats, to maintain a stable blood sugar level. Find what works for you - how much protein, carbs and fats should be included at each meal for optimal health. Talk to a healthcare professional.
- Complex carbohydrates are found in sweet potatoes, legumes, beans, and brown rice. It is recommended to be eaten in moderation or according to your fitness goals.
- Eat balanced meals/snacks to include: complex carbohydrates, protein and essential fats according to your body weight and activity level.
- Your body chemistry changes with age; therefore, you should continually monitor and adjust your lifestyle habits accordingly.
- Keep a food journal. Make a decision to start with one change weekly or monthly if that works better for you - remember this is a marathon not a sprint. List what complex carb you chose to substitute for simple carbs and the date. Write down how you felt each week after you implemented the change. Did you notice any physiological changes? Did you sleep better? Did you have more energy? Did you have fewer cravings?
- Set short-term goals rather than giving up all unhealthy, bad, or unproductive habits at once. Start with any of the items

we have discussed above or come up with another one. Start with a day, then work up to two weeks and so on.

- Make a decision to give up something that is harming your health. Pick 2-3 foods or drinks to wean off and start with 1 day, progressing to 3 days, 7 days, 2 weeks, 30 days, 60 days, and so on. You will have cravings and withdrawals and that is to be expected; practice self-control in order to make progress.
- Do not bring foods that you want to avoid into the house under any circumstance. Once it's in the house, you are more likely to eat it. If your excuse is that it's for the kids, keep in mind if it is affecting you negatively, how will it affect them? As with any addiction, the cravings and the desire for that food will eventually subside. Stop giving into the negative behaviors and find alternative solutions. Instead of a cookie, eat an apple with almond butter.
- Going cold turkey is not for everyone. As you make changes, give the mind time to catch up with what the body is now doing. Once you are consistently giving your body the nutrients it needs, the cravings will begin to dissipate. Trust me, it took me almost a year before I stopped having soda cravings.
- A trick to suppress cravings and work past the withdrawals: reduce stress, do an activity that takes your mind off that desire; this does not include watching TV - instead, read a book or magazine. Other options include brushing your teeth, drinking water with lemon/lime, adding some peppermint leaves and cucumber to it; eat a handful of nuts; or if it is not too late in the evening, have a small piece of fruit. Physical activity also works - take a walk or run outside especially during good weather.
- Eat smaller portioned meals and snacks; eat in moderation throughout the day, do not starve yourself.
- Your biggest meal should be lunch or very early dinner.

- Eat a light dinner or snack at least 2-3 hours prior to bedtime. This could be one slice of sprouted bread with almond butter and a small amount of fruit preserves or hummus and celery sticks. Remember, if the last meal is at 5 p.m. and your next meal is not until 7 a.m. the following morning, that means 14 hours or more without eating, and your body is probably already in starvation mode and storing fat.

We live in a busy world and lead hectic lives. Many of us desire convenient and easy ways to make our lives less stressful. Unfortunately, because of the way our food is manufactured today, we have to make certain that we are educating ourselves to make informed decisions and better lifestyle choices. In doing so, it may not seem that balanced meals or intentional eating is the easier way, but it is the better way to maintain good health and prevent diseases. Make a decision today to change something that is potentially harming your health.

SHOCKING FACT: Any form of diabetes may have risk factors that include, but are not limited to, kidney failure, blindness, amputation, high blood pressure, heart problems and much more. New research shows that belly fat, brain memory problems, Alzheimer's, and autoimmune disease may be considered the new type 3 diabetes.

CHAPTER 13

Secret Four: Get Movin' - Build Habits Not Equipment

On The Move

"Chains of habit are too light to be felt until they are too heavy to be broken."
- Warren Buffett

Decisions, Decisions

Every day we make decisions on what and how much to eat, or whether we have time to work out. The number one reason people say they do not work out is the same reason for not cooking - a lack of time. Over time, we become frustrated, unmotivated, and surrender to the busyness of work and family matters. We begin to lose sight of what it means to have fun every day and to truly live. Instead, we live for the next big vacation or the once a week trip to the gym or Zumba class. We lose the carefree ways of childhood play from our everyday living. More than likely, we lose interest in physical activity because we forget the connection between fun and movement that we felt as children; rigid schedules and obligations replace fun and movement. Therefore, prioritizing physical activity (playing) becomes less important, and it begins to feel more like a chore and less like fun. Why do we lose sight of something that is so essential to our health and brings us joy? Do we stop the desire to have fun, or are we caught in a rut? I am more inclined to say we are caught in a rut and the rat race of this thing called life. We lose focus that physical activity is more exhilarating than sitting in front of the TV. We do not lose the desire to have fun because many of us continue to engage with friends and attend social events periodically. Therefore, it's not that we do not want "fun," we trick the mind into believing that something is only fun if it does not require much physical activity.

Physical Activity and the Brain

Many of us become accustomed to sitting behind a desk all day without much movement. Due to our hunter and gatherer DNA, humans need physical activity. When we are not moving regularly, our cells become oxygen deficient. Movement creates deep breathing and elevated heart rate; as a result, oxygen capacity is increased to the cells and the entire body revitalizes. Over time, a lack of physical activity can have a negative impact on your brain, health, and overall quality of life. Have you ever heard the saying, "You think better on your feet"? It is actually a proven fact. The brain becomes active when the body is in motion due to increased blood flow and oxygen, which creates more stimulation, releases endorphins, and improves brain function. If you feel tired and fatigued, it could be due to a lack of physical activity and oxygen deprived cells.

When you are *not* physically active, you are more likely to suffer depression, heart disease, diabetes, high blood pressure, high cholesterol, hormonal imbalance, memory loss, and arthritis. According to the Parkinson Disease Foundation, exercise has been known to improve other issues such as memory loss, Parkinson's, and Alzheimer's. There are so many benefits to physical activity if we just push through, get off the sofa, find a physical activity you enjoy and start building new habits.

Regular physical activity has been proven to display the following benefits:

- Increased chances of living longer
- Improved self-image and confidence
- Reduced depression
- Enhanced energy level
- Improved mobility
- Increased muscle and bone strength
- Improved quality of sleep

An article written by Fitness and Exercise says, about a third of New Year's resolvers make weight loss their primary goal, and about 15% aim to begin an exercise program. Most people "fall off the treadmill" because they say, "I am too tired, too busy, it's too boring, or too hard." A U.S. government survey shows that 75% of people will keep their resolution for a week; 64% of the remaining last for a month; and only 46% of the remaining will ever make it to the six-month mark.

My desire is for you to be a part of the 46% and one way of achieving that is to address the root cause of the problem. Why did you stop working out in the first place? What is your real intrinsic motivation to start again? What is the fear of not wanting to become active? Remember, without goals and motivation, your aspirations often fall by the wayside. Your motivation should not just be to look good and lose weight for your class reunion. That becomes a temporary external reason and usually does not create permanent habits. Les Brown said it best, *"Wanting something is not enough. You must hunger for it. Your motivation must be absolutely compelling in order to overcome the obstacles that will invariably come your way."* In Secret One, we discussed managing the stresses in your life, developing self-importance, and setting goals. Physical activity is one of those things we should prioritize to achieve stress management, alone time and improve self-esteem. Ask yourself the hard questions: How are you training your brain to perform a new behavior? How do you perceive physical activity? What is preventing you from engaging in physical activity? Be open and honest with yourself; this will help you move forward and overcome those barriers.

Love the Rain

As children, many of us were encouraged to get outside and play. Whether running around, playing catch, jumping rope, or kicking a ball, it was physical activity and it was fun. I particularly enjoyed running around the yard in the rain. I do not know why that made me happy, but it did. As a teenager, my mother encouraged me to stay active; we routinely engaged in water or step aerobics classes, and took family walks after dinner.

As the obligations and responsibilities of adulthood took over, I re-prioritized my activities, which meant that working out and participating in physical activity went on the back burner. As with many individuals, I perceived it as hard work and a burden to my schedule. At the time, I did not realize, understand or correlate the true benefits it added to my health; in turn, I allowed everything else to take priority. When I did go to the gym, it was spontaneous and unfulfilling. I did not spend time in the moment, de-stressing or enjoying my time alone. I was usually "too busy" thinking about all my other responsibilities or feeling guilty about not spending time with my daughter, which defeated the purpose of being there.

Day after day, year after year, I continued to put working out on my "to do" list, but I was not making any progress on that goal, because life kept getting in the way - or so I thought. After more than eight years of inconsistency, gaining about 20-30 pounds, and still battling blood sugar issues, something had to change in my life, but I did not know how to go about it. I thought I was doing all I could do; I had about a 40% healthy diet, but the pounds were still adding on, I thought it was just a normal part of aging. Until John's "back fat" comment, I did not attribute my circumstances to a lack of exercise or bad eating habits.

I worked diligently over the years to change my eating habits, cooking at home and cutting back drastically on the processed foods. I eradicated my soda and candy addiction, and I was working on ending the nightly pastry addiction. I was doing some form of exercise at least 2-3 days per week, but mostly weights with very little cardiovascular exercise; I did not like running because it was boring. Therefore, I did not try anything that resembled running or any form of cardio to increase my heart rate. I had to come to terms with the fact that the extra weight and inches were not an issue of my appearance, but, more importantly, a sign that my health was still in jeopardy. The increasing size of my mid-section was a sure sign of not only stress, but also poor eating habits and lack of activity. I was just at the beginning of this journey and had more adjustments to make for continual improvements. The information John and the trainer shared gave me hope that I could not only change my health issues, but that I did not have to accept my weight gain as part of the aging process (see Chapter 12).

Can't Fool Physics

Initially, my brain avoided the cardiovascular exercise because I thought it was "hard" and I did not like it. I tried some no-carb diets and diet pills, but those did not work for me either. I did not become serious about exercise until I failed at the no-carb diet and I met a personal trainer who confirmed that I needed to incorporate consistent cardiovascular training, not just to lose the inches, but to achieve many other health benefits as well. With this, the question then became, how do I make the process something fun and enjoyable, and without neglecting my other responsibilities?

I got creative and found ways to include my daughter by enrolling her in swimming classes at the YWCA. During her sessions, I used my newfound love - the elliptical and StairMaster - at the gym. Afterwards, we spent additional time in the pool where I swam laps and played with her. We raced each other and she thought it was fun and playful. She practiced her swimming techniques, while keeping me physically active and, honestly, I loved it and I relished our time together. It allowed me to spend time engaging with her outside of homework or chores. I felt young, vibrant and energized. When I made physical activity fun and enjoyable, it felt less difficult and more interesting than previously thought. The feeling of a good sweat became exhilarating. My trainer developed high-intensity interval training (HIIT) workouts for me to do at home or outside, so I alternated those with the elliptical and StairMaster and I did not have to incorporate any form of running to get my cardio. I found little things to entertain myself to make it exciting in order to continue working out. I listened to music on my Walkman (we did not have iPods back then) and I got in a zone for 20-30 minutes. I loved the time alone to clear my mind and work on my health. Currently, I still follow this same regimen, finding various activities that interest me. Recently, I tried stand-up paddle boarding; it was hard work, but I love being on the water so that kept my interest.

Summer Love

During the summer months, I incorporated going to the park with my daughter. We played on the swings, ran around, and even played on the monkey bars; we took walks, raced each other, biked or speed walked. Additionally, I formed a power walk group at work, which I took advantage of for a half hour during lunch break, two days per week. I purchased workout videos to add some variety. I accepted my ADHD personality and realized that in order to keep things interesting, I had to change them up; when doing the same routine repeatedly, I grow bored, and would lose interest and stop doing it.

In this regard, I surrounded myself with options and planned accordingly. Being actively involved in a fun loving way with my daughter made us both happier, and I saw positive changes in her behavior. I was more involved with her in a playful manner, not merely dropping her off at swim class or gymnastics, or watching her on the playground, and she loved it. Furthermore, I felt less stressed and I did not feel guilty for leaving her to workout anymore.

Michelle's Proud Moment

During our last weekly call of 12 sessions, my client Michelle expressed that she was impressed and proud of how far she had come in just 12 short weeks. She then shared an incident she had with a friend who had visited after they'd not seen each other in almost a year. She explained when she last saw her friend she described her as being a "little tiny thing, about 110 to 120 pounds with an athletic build, who used to run." Now the friend had gained about 40 to 50 pounds, she had acne and did not look as vibrant as before. The friend admitted that she was not working out as much as prior to getting married, and that her eating habits had changed drastically. Michelle could not believe that her friend had experienced such a drastic physical change within such a short time.

The friend visited during Michelle's walk time, instead of dismissing the friend or not sticking to her plan to walk, Michelle invited her friend to walk with her, and she accepted. Side note: I was so proud of Michelle, because prior to my involvement, which she admitted, the friend's visit would have been a perfect excuse for her not to do her walk, if she went at all. She knew that she had to keep on task and not get back into her old habits. Michelle stated during the walk that they had to stop a few times, because the friend seemed to have problems keeping up and was not breathing properly. Michelle said, "I was completely flabbergasted at this point." She could not understand how this could have happened especially for a person who had been so physically active and loved running. She also could not understand how she herself took the walk without any problems when she had only started brisk walking about three weeks prior.

Prior to working with me, Michelle did not participate in any sort of workout or cardiovascular activity on a regular basis. She'd had a gym membership for over three years and admittedly only used it a few times. She did not have diabetes or high blood pressure, but she did have severe digestive problems and she was hospitalized a couple times due to bowel obstruction; per her healthcare provider, she is overweight and she admitted to poor eating habits.

Set Small Goals

When clients start my program, they are enlightened with information that they have not previously heard. They become excited to discover how easy it could be to change poor eating habits, get on the road to better health, and lose weight. We individualize the path to accomplish your goals, which includes starting in small increments. If that means making a commitment three days a week to walk for one minute - yes, I said a minute - that is what we will do; it must be a realistic goal. Walking for a minute may sound ridiculous but it makes the goal more realistic and attainable. Once you get into the habit, it makes it easier for you to build upon that success and feel accomplished.

During the program, weighing yourself is discouraged; many people become frustrated and distracted by the fluctuation of the scale - muscle weighs more than fat. Initially you will lose water and fat weight, and you will begin to build muscle. You may not see much of a difference on the scale, as muscle weighs more than fat, but you will notice how your clothes fit more loosely. You will begin to gain more energy, and better sleep; aches and pains will start to dissipate. Once you realize that even though you do not see a difference on the scale, especially after your first 10-20 pounds of water weight was easily lost, you begin to attain other benefits and agree that the scale can be deceiving, discouraging and frustrating. Keep in mind this is not a weight loss program - it's a lifestyle change. If you attend to the inside, you will see the transformation on the outside.

Physical activity, also referred to as exercise and working out, can reduce the risk of developing diabetes and other health concerns as well as improve your health and overall quality of life. Physical activity and exercise can have significant, immediate and long-term health benefits. If you have not been active, my suggestion is to start by building up the habit; get into the practice of simply moving before enrolling full-time in a gym or buying home equipment. Many of us run out, buy equipment, and join a gym, but motivation quickly wanes and all of it goes unused. Instead, look at buying equipment or joining a gym as a reward or a progression of your commitment. You do not need equipment to get started.

Make a decision to get active and then practice the physical movements to avoid injury. This is extremely important because it is very easy to injure yourself if you are not using proper form while exercising. There are four basic movements that will help strengthen the body and support health: push-ups, pull ups, planks and squats. Do these exercises at home, in the park, at work or at the gym. The only equipment you need is already in your possession: a plan, your brain and your body. Make sure to speak with your medical practitioner before you start any form of exercise or physical activity.

Habits First, Equipment Later

Tips to Build Habits First, Equipment Later

AT WORK

- Get up and move at least every hour. Post reminder notes in places where you have a tendency to sit without much movement for an extended time, i.e. your desk.
- Set your clock to get up and move around at least once every hour for 5 minutes.
- Take a brisk walk to the restroom or get some water. If you work in a multi-level building, go up and down a couple flights of stairs. Take the stairs instead of elevator. Even if you go halfway and take the elevator the remainder of the way, it's okay.
- Do 2-3 sets of 10 to 12 push-ups using the edge of your desk; increase reps as you begin to master the movements and build endurance. Do the same of any of the other movements. Do as many reps as you can and move quickly.
- While you are talking on the phone, stand instead of sitting and do chair squats, when possible.

- Do lunges at your desk. If you are in a cubicle, do not worry about others around you – they will soon follow. Be a leader.
- Take a power walk outside, weather permitting, or inside during your lunch break. Do it 15 to 20 minutes before you eat.
- Do yoga stretches or poses at your desk or the break room.

AT HOME

- Post reminder notes in places where you have a tendency to sit without much movement for an extended time. Posting it on the TV screen is usually an excellent place.
- Say "NO" to screen time and "YES" to playtime.
- Get outside and play games with the kids: shoot hoops, throw the football or Frisbee, play hopscotch, kick a soccer ball, or jump rope. Just get moving.
- Stop at the park or recreational center on your way home from work for a 20-30 minute workout a couple times a week. This will help you to de-stress and calm your spirit before going home.
- Do chores: rake the leaves, mow the lawn, clean the house while dancing, or walk the dog with the children.
- Put in a yoga or other workout DVD (or YouTube video) even when you do not feel like it - just show up. You will love yourself for it afterwards.
- Do walking lunges around house. Master the move to avoid injury and do not rush through the movements. Remember quality over quantity.
- Find a line-dance mix online or on YouTube and dance for 15 to 20 minutes.
- Remember something is better than nothing! Even if you have 5 minutes a few times throughout the day.
- Find an *accountability* partner. This is a huge aspect of being successful as a beginner. *"Find a friend and work out with them"* - Tony Horton.

- Do an enjoyable activity. Venture out and try new things, even things you think you will not enjoy or are afraid of trying. It gives you the opportunity to find a variety of physical activity you enjoy. It is important to change up the movements and routines in order to cause muscle confusion.
- Instead of giving yourself a reason not to get active, give reasons why you should. Physical activity can be accomplished with or without weights in places other than in a gym.
- Mark your calendar when you do any form of physical activity. It's like giving yourself a gold star for being active. It reminds you that you did an activity, and, in turn, you feel accomplished, thus increasing your motivation.

KEEP A JOURNAL: Be accountable to yourself!

- List the activities you did each day. The best way to remember something is to write it down.
- Track how long were you engaged in the activity.
- Did you have a set time or was it spontaneous? When you plan a time to workout it sets you up for success.
- How did you feel after each workout?
- Did you notice any physiological changes throughout the week?
- It's important to stretch your muscles before and after a session.

SHOCKING FACT: Regular exercise is a complex multi-faceted behavior that exercise professionals and scientists need to explain in order to help clients stay active, while keeping it simple and becoming healthier. Research suggests that 50% of those starting an exercise program will drop out within the first 6 months, Wilson and Brookfield, 2009. Usually, this is not due to a lack of motivation; it is due to a lack of understanding, and the level of difficulty and intensity of the program. This leaves the individual feeling frustrated and ashamed. The goal of creating habits is to create long-lasting behavioral change. Make a commitment, get into a habit, set a goal, do not give up, and you will create long-lasting behavioral change that will stimulate the body; you will begin to crave the "good stuff."

CHAPTER 14

Variety is the Spice of Life

"*Genius (success) is 1% inspiration and 99% perspiration.*" - Thomas Edison

Mis-education

Exercise does not have to be time-consuming and excruciating in order to be effective. For the average person, a good fitness program consists of exercises that work the entire body and cardiovascular system. Weight-bearing, weight-resistance or strength exercises enhance the function and health of the bones, muscles, joints, and connective tissues, whereas cardiovascular activities improve the function and health of the heart, lungs, and blood vessels.

A common misconception is that these two forms of exercise must be performed separate to achieve maximum results. Some exercise trainers add to the myth and misunderstanding, promoting the idea that intense cardio burns and assists with weight loss while weight-bearing methods gain muscles. These opinions leave most individuals in a dilemma, not knowing the benefits or how to incorporate both methods simultaneously to decrease workout time and maximize results. Be cautious; entering a catabolic state, burning muscle for fuel, can happen when you are not practicing appropriate physical activities. A catabolic state usually occurs when exercising at a high intensity level for more than 45 minutes daily or on an empty stomach. Innately, when your body is in this constant high level, it believes it is in "fight or flight" or stress mode. The body begins to release a "fat storing" hormone known as cortisol in order to protect itself. In addition, excessive insulin production is stimulated and deactivates the genes that promote efficient fat burning. In essence, you are reversing the intended goal to burn fat and lose weight.

For some, it can be discouraging and we decide not to work out because commercials and infomercials affirm high-intensity workouts as the best way to attain weight loss, or we see athletes performing at a high intensity and sweating profusely, and think this is how we should workout. These types of workouts are typically conducted with the guidance of a professional. Personal trainer Jonathan Ross, ACE, NSCA, says such high-intensity workouts are done only by a very small percentage of the population. There is a connection between exercise and pain, discomfort, and soreness - but it does not mean all workouts must be excruciating to gain results.

Combining balance, strength and cardiovascular training with healthy dietary habits is highly recommended for achieving better and faster results, and preventing muscle loss. Adding an all-out intensive cardio session, such as interval sprints for 15-20 minutes per week is ideal to accomplish your wellness goal. Once you build the habit to get moving and increase your understanding of physical activity, the transformation can now begin. The workout approach should be individualized based on body type and goals. It's important to seek professional assistance to ensure you are on the right track. Proper weight training will increase the strength and endurance of your muscles, which will improve your cardiovascular efficiency and burn more calories and fat in the process. The two approaches should complement rather than compete with each other. This method of training keeps the body burning fat even after the workout is completed.

You Do Not Have to Run a Marathon

To get the brain and muscles stimulated, research suggests that exercise is ideally performed just outside of your comfort zone. Jonathan Ross says, "You're taking your body a little outside where it is because it needs that challenge - that stimulus - to be able to improve." It's important to get active and get moving; raking leaves, cleaning the house or a brisk walk is considered effective exercise. A rule of thumb, stated by various studies - achieve aerobic heart rate at least three times a week. Aerobic exercise is reaching a heart rate of 50% - 75% of your resting rate. Anaerobic exercise is anything above 85% of your resting heart rate, and should be achieved at least one time in 7-10 days lasting 30-60 minutes.

Knowing your heart-rate training zone benefits everyone from the beginning exerciser trying to lose weight or get lean, to the highly conditioned athlete. If you're not using this technique, you are more than likely not achieving your goal. The key to success is to elevate your heart rate into the correct training zone, so your effort matches your goals. If checking your heart rate manually is too troublesome, it may be a good idea to invest in a heart monitor.

To determine your heart rate, the University of Colorado researchers suggest the following formula. Keep in mind, this method does not take into account your fitness level or inherited genes, which can make your true maximum heart rate 10 to 20 beats per minute higher or lower than the age-predicted number.

Here are six easy-to-follow steps that will help you calculate your ideal heart-rate training zone.

1. Determine your resting heart rate (RHR) - Before getting out of bed in the morning or before getting in bed, find your pulse either on the wrist or the neck, set a timer, count the number of beats per 10 second (bps), and multiple by 6 for your RHR. For example 11 bps x 6 = 66. Do this for several consecutive days to get a consistent reading.

2. Calculate your Maximum Heart Rate (MHR) - Subtract your age from 220. The result is an age-predicted maximum beats per minute. For example 220 - 47 (age) = 172 (MHR).
3. Calculate your Heart-Rate Reserve - Subtract your heart's resting rate from your maximum heart rate. For example 172 – 66 = 106 heart rate reserves.
4. Calculate your Aerobic Training Heart-Rate Range - For fat burning this range will lie between 50% and 75% of your heart-rate reserve as calculated in step 3. Using the example above, 50% of 106 beats per minute = 53 and 75% of 106 = 74. Next, add your resting heart rate to both numbers separately: 53 + 66 = 119 and 74 + 66 = 140. Your heart rate during aerobic training for a 47 year old will most efficiently burn fat at 119 to 140 beats per minute.
5. Calculate your Aerobic (vigorous exercise) Training Heart-Rate Range - The range to achieve maximum fitness endurance is between 75% and 85% of your heart - rate reserves. Follow the same directions as above using 75% and 85%.
6. Calculate your Anaerobic Heart Rate - This rate represents the upper limits of aerobic for improved athletic performance. Follow the same formula in step # 4 using 85% - 100% for your heart rate reserves.

It is important to know your target heart rate to determine aerobic (fat burning) or anaerobic training and stay within that zone for at least 30-45 minutes to achieve ideal results. For the sake of simplicity, aerobic refers to how the muscle cells contract repeatedly without fatigue. Anaerobic metabolism can impair muscle contractions causing fatigue. The body typically enters into an aerobic state between 50% and 75% of the resting rate. At 50% of your max heart rate, the body burns a ratio of 60% fat to 40% glycogen (sugar stored for energy in the muscles and liver). At 75% of your max heart rate, the ratio is 35% fat to 65% glycogen, and at even higher intensities, the ratio of fat to glycogen is even lower.

Once per week, interval sprints or other forms of interval training should be conducted at above 85% of your heart rate for optimal results. You can accomplish this goal even with interval training. Of course, check with your healthcare practitioner before starting any exercise program.

Change is Good

As my daughter became older, I thought about other creative ways to stay active where she could remain involved. We both enjoyed the bonding time and it allowed us to stay active while doing it. Going to the gym on a regular basis was not my cup of tea, and still is not. I like variety and change of scenery, especially the outdoors. During her extracurricular activities where I could not interact directly with her, I used that time to work out. When she had track practice, I used the field and bleachers for my workout. During her dance classes, I went to an outside area or used one of their empty rooms. To prevent boredom and stagnation, creating a variety of activities is best of me.

Ordinarily, I planned time to work out, but did not always plan the activity until that day. I work out according to how I feel, keeping in mind to exercise various muscle groups. Every few months I changed the routine, location and/or scenery. I alternated activities such as biking, rollerblading, yoga, Pilates, PiYo, running or hiking and incorporated 2-3 days of high intensity interval training. Periodically, I hired a personal trainer or joined a boot camp to learn new methods and techniques to later implement on my own. Due to the accessibility of the Internet, there is no reason you cannot find a good workout plan at a much lower cost than joining a gym. There are many online sites to download a variety of workout routines free of charge or at minimal cost.

At some point, you may choose to invest in group fitness, gym membership, or a personal trainer. There are various options at your disposal; you must find the ones that work for you instead of making excuses for not working out. I suggest starting with building momentum, getting into the habit, and then taking that leap. Many people try to rationalize by saying, "If I am paying for it, I will go and it will encourage me." Just remember, research shows that only 18% of gym membership seekers actually utilize it.

Brenda's Running a Marathon

Brenda was overweight according to her doctor's diagnosis. She had a long-standing gym membership that she only used when I went with her. Prior to meeting me, she rarely used it. She stated she initially signed up to encourage her ten-year-old granddaughter, who has also considered overweight, to exercise. Brenda's motivation was her granddaughter, and not her own health. Her intentions were great, but her motive was not meaningful enough, and, more than likely, she would not be successful until it became so. After four weeks on the 12-week program, Brenda was encouraged to find a reliable accountability partner to workout with her. She was no longer doing it for her granddaughter; she was doing it because she knew she had to do something to change her health status in order to be around for her granddaughter and to be a role model to her. Initially, she did simple outside activities until she decided she wanted to utilize the gym again. Several times, other family members accompanied her; based on her initiative they followed.

One day, she called me completely excited and wanted to share what she accomplished. She said, "You will never guess what I did." Brenda began to explain with excitement, "I ran, I ran. I was walking for a few minutes on the treadmill as we discussed, and as I have been doing over the last few weeks and I began to slowly increase my speed. I had music on and got into a zone. The next thing I knew, I was running, but the great thing was I did not realize I was running until I stopped. My Mom was walking on the treadmill next to me and she said, 'Do you know what you just did?'" She said, "I didn't until now, and it feels great." Brenda explains that this is something she never thought she would do. She thought she would not like running. She thought her back and knee would hurt or give out due to her weight, but that did not happen. After several weeks of continuing and slowly increasing her goals, she decided she wanted to run a marathon within the next four months. After discussing her goals, we decided it is best to set this goal in small steps for success. Four months was probably a little too ambitious and not realistic only because I knew Brenda's history and personality, so we agreed a year would be a more realistic goal. I introduced her to a local women's running group at no cost, so she could get in that mind frame and start training. They participated in 3K-5K runs, and later got her involved with a local chapter to begin additional training.

Brenda saw great changes in her eating habits, health and overall lifestyle. She is now sleeping better and feels she has a more peaceful attitude about life. She is still running with the group, but has not increased yet to a half marathon, which is okay; it is about taking one step at a time and being consistent. She is involved in various physical activities that she enjoys, and are beneficial to her overall health.

Feel Empowered

As a child, I was not involved with organized sports, so when John suggested we join a volleyball team to add variety to our workout routine, I felt intimidated. I doubted my athletic abilities and did not want to embarrass myself. The volleyball team was made up of complete strangers who randomly signed up at a local recreation center and played every Friday night just for fun. These individuals were ordinary people who ranged from average athletic ability to none at all. They were individuals who wanted physical activity, enjoyed the game and wanted the camaraderie. After observing John at a few of the games, I realized there was no reason to feel intimidated; it was more about having "pure" fun and less about competition. I eventually joined and loved it. No one became upset if I missed a few hits; they were all supportive, not only to me, but to each other. I built up the courage and tried something I never thought I would, and actually became somewhat good at it. We looked forward to the camaraderie every Friday evening.

Keeping physical activity fresh, entertaining, and enjoyable is important to maintaining one's interest for most individuals. Adding variety to your workout can also keep you motivated. It is great for the body, because it creates muscle confusion, allowing muscles that may not be used in one activity to become involved in another. Muscle confusion is great for brain stimulation - when we get bored, our brain becomes bored too, and it wants stimulation. Remember from the previous chapter, a body in motion creates brain stimulation.

With consistency and a little effort, your body can and will change. It is up to you to define what that transformation will look like. Below I have outlined various methods of physical activity and how it affects your body for maximum improvement. This information was taken from Health Science Academy course work materials.

- *Aerobic activities* make you breathe harder and your heart beat faster. Aerobic activities can be moderate or vigorous in their intensity. For moderate activities (15 to 30 minutes), you can talk while you do them, but not have lengthy conversations. Examples include line or ballroom dancing, brisk walks, shoveling snow, water aerobics, active gardening, or actively playing with the children. For vigorous activities (10 to 15 minutes), you can only say short phrases without stopping to catch your breath. Examples are running, swimming, race-walking, cycling, fast dancing, or jogging.
- *Muscle-strengthening activities* make your muscles stronger. These exercises can be done with or without weight or resistance bands. These gravity-resistant moves involve having the muscles work against a force or weight. This can be achieved with exercise like push-ups, sit-ups, lunges, squats, lifting weights, and working with resistance bands. You can play a good game of tug-of-war, swing on the monkey bars, or rock climb. It is important to work all the different parts of the body - your legs, hips, back, chest, stomach, shoulders, and arms. The mid to lower torso is the powerhouse of the body.

Working the legs helps give support to the back and abdomen.
- *Bone-strengthening activities* make the bones stronger, preventing osteoporosis and improving bone density. They include jumping rope, jumping jacks, running, brisk walking, tennis, basketball, hopping, skipping, jumping, and volleyball. These activities and exercises are especially important for children and adolescents to do as they are still growing and developing. These activities produce a force on the bones that promotes bone growth and strength.
- *Balance and stretching activities* enhance physical stability and flexibility, which reduces the risk of injuries and increases balance when doing any activity. These will include gentle stretching, dancing, Pilates, yoga, martial arts, and tai chi.

There are various types of training such as plyometrics and high intensity interval training that encompass any combination of the above techniques to give you optimal results in a shorter period of time.

Below are a list of low to moderate exercises. It gives you examples for exercises in the appropriate category and number of calories burned. The calories burnt chart is just for your knowledge. I suggest to my clients to focus on the heart rate and eating habits to measure progress. Just think, if you ate an 8 oz bag of potato chips - that's 1,217 calories. It's impossible to burn that off in 30 minutes. Therefore, exercise alone will not help you lose weight. The goal of exercising is about maintaining and achieving healthy bones, building muscle, and a life free from health concerns.

The content below is referenced from the Health Science Academy course materials.

Aerobic Exercises - Low Exercise

Calories Burned

	130 LBS.	180 LBS.	230 LBS.
Walking (3.0 mph)	103	142	184
Cleaning (vigorous)	133	184	235
Mowing lawn (push mower)	163	225	288
Cycling (10-11.9 mph)	177	245	313
Ballroom dancing (fast)	163	225	288
Golf, pulling clubs	147	203	206
Swimming (leisurely)	177	245	313
Aerobics (low-impact)	147	203	260
Calisthenics (beginner's yoga)	133	184	235
Racquetball (casual)	207	287	366

Aerobic Exercises - Vigorous Exercise

Calories Burned

	130 LBS.	180 LBS.	230 LBS.
Jogging	207	287	366
Running (12 min. mile)	235	326	416
Hiking (rigorous)	177	245	313
Shoveling snow	177	245	313
Basketball	235	326	416
Tennis (singles	235	326	416
Skiing (cross-country)	265	367	470
Cycling (12-13.9 mph)	235	326	416
Aerobics (high impact)	207	287	366
Calisthenics (vigorous, push-ups)	235	326	416

Physical activity is important, and many of these activities cost little to no money. For many years, I was a single parent, living on a social worker's budget. The phrase "no cost or free" was my best friend and I signed up for almost any physical activity that was free. I urge you, if not for yourself, to be a good example for your children. The more they see you being active, the more active they will want to be now and as they grow. Take the habits you have started and make a commitment to do some form of physical activity for 30 days. When you make a commitment to yourself and make it known to others, you are more likely to hold yourself responsible.

"Half of life is showing up." - Woody Allen

Below are some tips to help you get physically active at little to no cost.

No Cost

- Take a hike in the woods, the mountains, or at a local park.
- Brisk walks, jogging, running, or bike riding.
- Playing with the children: Tug of war, tag football, running around.
- Cleaning the house.
- Gardening or yard work: weeding, raking, shoveling snow
- Join a softball or volleyball team.
- Jump Rope - You don't need a rope, you can pretend.
- Swimming at local community pools - great form of exercise and one of the best cures for body pain.
- Explore a variety of workout programs free, online or on social media sites such as Instagram and Pinterest.
- Try a variety of floor exercises: Push-ups, jumping jacks, lunges, squats, and abdominals crunches. Many of these can be done at your desk or break-room.

Little Cost

- Indoor rock climbing, many places charge a minimal fee.
- Zumba classes are a great cardiovascular workout.
- Boot camp classes offer beginner to advanced levels; so don't be intimidated to try.
- Aerobic swimming.
- Learn to play tennis; local parks or community recreation centers.
- Yoga, PiYo or Pilates, or Insanity - either a live class, DVD or online.
- StairMaster, treadmill, elliptical, stationary bike.
- Invest in a stability ball; most come with a CD or DVD with a variety of exercises.
- Short on time? Try shorter (15 to 20 minutes), very intensive interval workouts.

SHOCKING FACT: Do not underestimate the benefits of Yoga or Pilates. They build flexibility, help create and define muscles, help with balance, relaxation and meditation. We need balance for everyday activity like walking around. Do not think you need to start with something very advanced in terms of running or weight lifting. The important thing is get moving, start on a schedule, stick to it (no excuses), and be active.

CHAPTER 15

Healthy is the New Sexy

"Health is like money, we never have a true idea of its value until we lose it."

- Josh Billings

Individuals regularly give up on exercise because they are not losing enough weight as fast as they'd like. Exercise alone won't result in weight loss; it's a combination of healthy eating habits and incorporating consistent physical activity. Recall from Secret One, 75%-80% of your body composition and health success is determined by how you eat. The foods you ingest determine hormonal manipulation and gene expression to increase the metabolism. Many individuals are involved in extreme workouts and still cannot seem to get rid of the excess body fat. There may be two convincing arguments; you are working outside of your fat burning zone and/or possibly dietary changes should be made.

The secrets discussed in this book all work hand-in-hand. Proper nutrition and stress management are an absolute necessity to give your body the fuel it needs in order to perform optimally. Consistent physical activity is needed to release the hormones necessary to maintain overall good health and quality of life. According to the CDC, consistent exercise and proper nutrition can help maintain a healthy weight and reduce the risk of cardiovascular disease, as well as lower risks for certain forms of cancer. The body needs quality fuel and proper maintenance to function optimally; nutrition and exercise help meet these requirements.

Avoid Empty Calories

Exercise, together with a proper diet, will help place your body in caloric deficit, which means you are burning more calories than you are consuming. Keep in mind that the body continues to burn calories and the metabolic system remains active even after intense physical activity. Eating foods high in nutritional value, but low in caloric content such as fresh fruit, cruciferous vegetables, and lean proteins such as fish and poultry, can also help keep the metabolic system active. The metabolic system helps the body receive the nutrition it needs without all the empty calories. It is important to eat at least 5-6 times per day using portion control; these are to include two to three snacks with a balanced portion of carbohydrates, essential fats, and protein; the ratio is determined by age and level of physical activity.

It is important to avoid or limit foods high in simple carbohydrates, i.e. simple sugar, and trans and saturated fats, as most are empty calories. A study from Clark University reveals that a diet high in cholesterol and "bad" fats can cause arterial plaque, a fatty deposit build up in the arteries, which slows blood circulation. Exercising regularly and reducing the fat and cholesterol intake will help fight plaque buildup.

Develop a Healthy Mindset

Consistent exercise can help improve your mental stability and support optimal cognitive function. According to the U.S. National Library of Medicine, exercise can reduce negative mental conditions such as anxiety, depression, and mood swings while improving self-esteem. Following the minimum recommendations for exercise - 15-30 minutes of aerobic training, 3-5 times per week as stated by the Department of Health and Human Services - can have tremendous benefits other than weight loss. It can improve alertness, analytical thinking and performance on the job, as well as the ability to perform minor tasks around the house.

Going to the gym for the sake of looking good or impressing someone is like going to Harvard to attain an associate degree. Although you may have good intentions with both - going to the gym or attending Harvard - you are not leveraging the full benefits of the tremendous resources they provide. In the past, when I worked out it was to keep in shape and look good. As soon as other life events came about, working out went on the back burner. Once motherhood and adult responsibilities increased, it became even less of a priority. Consequently, I shifted to working out only when it was convenient, when I felt like it and in my spare time, which seemed to be on rare occasions. I had a new "healthy" guy in my life and wanted to impress him and that effort to workout ended up being short-lived too. Despite my poor eating habits and inconsistent physical involvement, I became frustrated when I did not see much change in my physical appearance. At the time, looking good was important, but understanding health was not a priority. Initially, I did not understand the health benefits of physical activity and healthy eating. Looking good is relative and it did not give me the motivation or determination to be consistent.

Physical activity only became important to me once I understood and acknowledged the internal health benefits after many years. I finally understood that exercise is more than what I looked like on the outside. It was only then that I bought into it and accepted the positive impact it could have on my blood sugar level and in preventing other health issues. Thereafter, being healthy became my internal motivation. I developed a different perspective about physical activity; I wanted to live a healthy life and have an active lifestyle as long as possible. That meant I needed to eat healthy as well as incorporate physical activity into my daily routine and be consistent to achieve this goal.

In order to make this permanent change in my life, it had to become a deep-rooted motivation; I developed the mindset that this was fun and not a chore. I began to prioritize this approach when I planned it as a daily routine and made it a part of "me time". I enjoyed and looked forward to having that time to relax, de-stress, and reflect. Days when I preferred sitting on the couch watching television as opposed to being involved with physical activity, I self-talked, convincing myself to exercise. I reminded myself of the importance to my physiological well-being and the exhilarating feeling afterwards; that became my motivation. Once you commit to that mindset, it becomes easier to stay consistent with physical activity.

I am human and do periodically allow other things to clutter my mind or get me down, and I lose the energy to workout. I make an honest effort to control those situations, immediately stop the chatter and do something even if it means simply walking or cleaning the house to be active. I force myself to get out the house and stop the excuses; after all, we are creatures of habit. It is truly surprising when I do not engage in physical activity for a couple days; aches and pains emerge, lethargy and moodiness sets in. I don't like feeling that way, and it forces me to get back into the swing of things.

Take It to The Next Level

Within the last few years, I decided to take my physical activity to the next level. As previously mentioned, working out was "me time", but honestly, that was only in words. I say that because during my workout, I took phone calls, text messages and emails from clients, family members, the kids, and sometimes socialized with others. I became distracted, it took me longer to finish, I gave it less effort and it was less enjoyable. I decided to set boundaries and my workout time truly became "me time"; it was my time to zone out and enjoy the moment. Now I do not answer phone calls, text messages, or respond to emails. On my workout days, my family was informed not to call or text me unless it was an emergency and I avoid talking to anyone around me until I am finished. When I approached it from that perspective, it made my workout so much easier and more enjoyable.

Getting healthy and staying healthy is challenging. Many people I speak with see it as a destination, and it is not; it is a journey. It's a life-long process of trial and error, and adjustments; it's a lifestyle change. As a person ages, the body chemistry changes and it becomes more important to stay active. It is important to be in tune with your body and know when changes occur, such as with your hormones, digestive system, metabolism, and stamina. This may result in you altering what you eat and adjusting your physical regimen. You may experience frustration initially; be patient with your body and keep setbacks to a minimum. You are on the right road to successfully feeling and looking better; just stay active and trust the process.

In order to capitalize on the complete benefits of and maximize your workouts, it is imperative you supply your body with adequate nutrients. When I experimented with a no carbs, high protein diet, it had a negative impact on my system. I was unable to maintain a stable blood sugar level or adequate energy level to fully participate in physical activities. Life challenges have taught me it is better to make "small" sacrifices now, than "bigger" ones later.

Avoid Reverse Damage

Research shows that many individuals start an exercise program without knowledge about the dangers or the benefits. It is just as crucial to know the benefits as well as the dangers in order to prevent reverse damage. The body has a great memory regardless of how long it has been since your last physical activity involvement; once you start to move, the body will begin to respond accordingly. The brain recognizes what is going on and begins to release protective proteins and hormones like endorphins. These endorphins tend to minimize the discomfort of exercise, blocking the feeling of pain and causing a feeling of euphoria.

At the same time when we exercise, the brain thinks it is in stress mode so it goes into fight-or-flight response. Due to the fight-or-flight response, it is important to keep workouts to no more than 45 to 60 minutes per session so that you do not over-stress the body. Reversal damage begins when the body is in constant, high intensity, and over exhaustive state. Professional athletes are knowledgeable and are trained on how to minimize this damage, but even they cannot continue at a high level of training indefinitely. Continuous, high intensity activity can be counterproductive. We typically think more is better, and that is not always the case.

Lack of proper nutrients also causes reverse damage. If your calorie intake is too low, the body will use its reserves for energy, depleting the body of its reserves and vital nutrients. It is the same effect as when starvation occurs. The reserved fat and protein the body needs for everyday living now becomes the energy supplier to get you through your workouts or daily living. The initial thought may be *yes that's good, because it's using up my stored fats,* but that's not how it works. The protein is taken from lean muscle mass and converted into glucose. The lean muscle is what you want to build, not take away from it. If you're not consuming enough daily nutritious calories, your metabolism will slow down, as it doesn't need to do as much work to break down carbs and proteins because there isn't enough of it. Bottom line - get rid of those old myths that starving yourself will cause you to lose weight.

Stop Counting Calories, Count Meals

It is typical for me to eat 3-4 small meals a day, every 2-3 hours, with my last meal or snack no less than two hours prior to bedtime. I do not practice calorie counting, but I do practice portion control, eating nutritious calories instead of empty, useless ones. Be sure to include good carbs, fats, and protein in each meal and snack. The only time I pay attention to calories is to decipher if they are empty calories or useless food versus nutritious food. Eating or grazing throughout the day ensures that the metabolism is getting a "workout" all day. Foods that help the metabolism stay active include avocado, herbal teas, fruit, lean meat, fish, eggs and dark chocolate. Also consider metabolism boosting ingredients such as cinnamon, garlic, water, chili peppers, and apple cider vinegar.

Eating a late meal or snack ensures that I am not in starvation mode when I wake up and I have sufficient energy to workout. It's best not to eat less than 2-3 hours before bedtime; this ensures the metabolism gets the opportunity to rest and restore during sleep mode. If you are hungry when you wake up, have a small serving of fruit and protein prior to your workout. Of course, if you are not working out in the morning, eat a full meal. Even if your morning meal is only a smoothie, ensure it includes protein and essential fats like nuts, hemp, flaxseeds, coconut oil, and complex carbs such as fruit or vegetables. Make it simple.

Consumption of natural proteins through food sources such as fish, nuts, legumes, eggs, chicken, quinoa is best for preventing muscle loss. If the body is not getting enough protein to build or repair muscles, it begins converting muscle mass to fuel. Therefore, you are losing muscle instead of building it. It is important to consume complex carbs as well. The body uses a dual fuel source (fat + glucose) to feed muscles during physical activity. Glucose comes from the carbs you eat so if you consume too many carbs, the body will convert excess glucose into fat and store it, which is what you do not want (see Chapter 2). It is critical to practice portion control and eat regularly balanced meals and snacks. If it becomes confusing to devise a healthy eating lifestyle, speak with a health and wellness consultant, coach, or natural healthcare practitioner who is knowledgeable in healthy eating.

Below are some tips to help you "Get Your Sexy Back and Keep It":

- Morning workouts are best and most effective on a slightly empty stomach. Start each morning with a sense of accomplishment; it leaves less room for excuses and inconsistency.
- For afternoon or evening workouts, eat at least two hours prior, giving the food ample time to digest properly without disturbance.
- Choose a workout time, when you have the most energy.
- Use physical activity as a stress reliever and "me time".
- Ensure you are eating complex carbohydrates and essential fats in moderation.
- Get at least 6-8 hours of sleep daily. The body, metabolism and brain recover and restore during sleep.
- Keep a positive mindset. Be inspired. Understand the main goal of physical activity is to gain better health, and losing weight will follow.
- Be creative with your activities. Diversification and enjoyment is key.
- Be consistent; include some form of physical activity in your routine, three to five days/week at moderate to high intensity.
- Make your workout plan fit your life.
- Maintain your relationship with a health and wellness professional. They can provide guidance, keep you on track, and be a great support system and accountability partner. The goal is to teach you how to fish, not give you a fish.
- Seek a professional trainer when you are ready to take it to the next level.
- Let's get a move on it - Challenge Time- find something that works for you and commit to it at least 15-30 minutes, 2-3 times a week for 30 days, no excuses. Let me know how you

are doing by posting your comments/questions/result to my Facebook page: www.facebook.com/parkerlifestyle.
- Commit to working out for the next three months - build upon the above tip, engaging in activities 3-5 times a week i.e. walking the stairs at work, biking or high intensity work out; anything but spending extensive time behind your desk or on the couch.
- Continue to improve upon the activities you enjoy. If you are biking for five minutes, increase the time, speed and/or the difficulty level of the bike trail. Change is good.
- Purchase complementary equipment: free weights, ankle or chest vest weights, stability ball, and resistance bands,
- Purchase a DVD to challenge yourself.
- Join a Zumba, Yoga, Pilates, PiYo Live, boot camp or other group fitness class. Hire a personal trainer to ensure you are maximizing your workouts.
- Be patient with yourself. It takes time to undo the damage that has been done.
- DO NOT - I repeat, DO NOT - compare yourself to others. We are all created differently. You cannot compare someone else's end results to your beginning.

SHOCKING FACT: Studies show that exercise reduces stress by increasing hormones that boost happiness. Through physical activity, you can improve self-esteem, feel happier, have less mood swings, be more productive, and improve your memory - along with a host of other benefits.

CHAPTER 16

Secret Five: Natural Healing

Natural Remedies - Herbs, Supplements, and Vitamins

"The doctor of the future will give no medicine but will interest his patients in the care of the human frame, in diet, and in the cause and prevention of disease."

- Thomas Edison

What are Supplements?

In 1994, congress passed the Dietary Supplement Health and Education Act (DSHEA). According to DSHEA, a dietary supplement is a product that is intended to supplement your nutrient consumption. It contains one or more dietary ingredients including vitamins, minerals, herbs or other botanicals, amino acids, and certain other substances found in the diet (such as enzymes and edible organ tissues and glandular), or their constituents in concentrates, metabolites, extracts, or any combination thereof. Supplements are intended to be taken orally, in tablet, capsule, liquid, powder, or, gel capsule form.

Dietary supplements are regulated as foods, rather than drugs, for purposes of the United States Federal Food, Drug, and Cosmetic Act

(FD&C Act) and their labeling must identify them as a dietary supplement. Whether it is regulated as a food, dietary supplement, or a drug depends on the intended purpose and use. Intended use is determined by claims made on a product's label, branding, advertising and test results evaluated in a clinical study. If a claim is made about the impact of a nutritional product on the diagnosis, cure, mitigation, treatment, or prevention of a disease or health related condition, the product will be regulated as a drug not a food.

The FDA does not consider the purpose of a study to be therapeutic if the study simply measures the effect of a nutritional product on the structure or function of the body or only examines the mechanism by which the product exerts its effect. For example, a study of a dietary supplement's effect on normal structure or function in humans (e.g., calcium's effect on bone mass) or a study characterizing the mechanism by which a dietary supplement acts to maintain such structure or function (e.g., fiber's effect on bowel regularity) would not need new dietary ingredient (NDI). By comparison, a study evaluating a dietary supplement's ability to prevent osteoporosis, treat diarrhea associated with antibiotic use, chronic constipation, or lower cholesterol, likely would need an NDI notification; hence the reason for the disclaimer throughout this book. Herbs have been used for thousands of years throughout the world for various ailments. Research has shown using various herbs and supplements can benefit our health. Due to regulation, stipulations and policy outlined by The Food and Drug Administration (FDA), the alternative health industry must exercise extreme caution regarding health claims.

Today healthcare professionals recommend supplements for our children starting at birth; I do not recall ever taking supplements as a child growing up in Trinidad. I do not recall taking them in my teenage years either. In fact, my first recollection of a healthcare professional or anyone suggesting supplements in my daily regimen was not until I became pregnant. They recommended a prenatal multivitamin; no information was given about why it was necessary.

I took them because it was "doctor's orders." I noticed a few changes occurred while taking them, like my hair and nails were growing and appeared healthier, and my skin was glowing. I thought it was all due to the pregnancy, not recognizing the vitamins could have had something to do with it. Call me young and naïve, but it's true. It was not until a few years later while researching when I discovered that multivitamins might have some perks when taken on a daily basis. So, without any further context, I naturally purchased my first vitamin supplement from the grocery store; I looked for the most reasonably priced item without regards for the ingredients. Unbeknownst to me, however, I was probably causing additional damage to my body due to the poor quality of the supplements. I was oblivious to the fact that all supplements are *not* created equal. Routinely, we do things at the suggestion of healthcare professionals without being informed or conducting our own research. It is important to research and ask questions before putting any medication or supplements into your body.

Herbs, vitamins and supplements are increasingly popular today and more information is readily available than prior years. It is paramount to be informed about the various brands and their quality before you take any supplement. How much is needed? How long to take them? Does the FDA regulate them? What is the difference between herbs and supplements? Which is more beneficial? All of these are legitimate questions. The FDA regulates most supplements, but not in the same manner as food or drugs, leaving manufacturers with more flexibility, to some extent. I am not advocating the government be involved in this industry nor am I suggesting their regulation makes the product a better quality. I am implying a lack of regulation can often lead to inconsistency, misrepresentation, and poor quality amongst the wide variety of products on the market. The downside to a lack of regulation or research is that anyone can make a product and the quality is uncharted. Individuals must research what they are ingesting and become acquainted with manufacturers that are more reputable; there are various supplement and vitamin rating websites that provide thorough reviews: multivitaminguide.org, consumerlab.com, or consumerreports.org. Unfortunately, in the supplement and vitamin world, higher quality products in most cases, usually equates to a higher price. In this case, it is not a good idea to go with a cheaper product because typically this means the quality of ingredients are also inferior. You do not want to put something into your body that is counterproductive - it becomes as useless as eating empty calories.

Vitamins and minerals are essential for normal cell function, growth, and development. It is important for everyone to have an overall strategy for how they will achieve adequate vitamin and mineral intakes via food, herbs or supplements. Your medical or natural healthcare practitioner should monitor this activity during annual visits at the minimum. There are guidelines on daily-recommended use published by the Department of Health and Human Services and the U.S. Department of Agriculture (USDA). These guidelines provide science-based advice to promote health and to reduce risk for chronic disease through diet and physical activity. They form the basis for food, nutrition education, and information programs.

What are Vitamins?

Vitamins consist of 13 essential compounds that each performs a fundamental role for total body function. The 13 essential vitamins are defined in two categories. The first is fat-soluble vitamins, which are stored in the body's fatty tissue, and consists of vitamins A, D, E, and K. The second group consists of nine water-soluble vitamins, which includes Biotin, Folate, Niacin (vitamin B3), Pantothenic acid, Thiamine (vitamin B1), Riboflavin (or vitamin B2, which works with the other B vitamins), Pyroxidine (vitamin B6), vitamin B12, and vitamin C (ascorbic acid). The body must use water-soluble vitamins immediately; any leftover leaves the body through urination. Vitamin B12 is the only water-soluble vitamin that can be stored in the liver for many years without being harmful. When the body is lacking appropriate levels of nutrients, it becomes deficient causing significant health problems.

Another Shocking Diagnosis

By 2008, I believed things were going great with my health. My diabetes was managed; my stress levels improved, and my overall health seemed great. Around late 2008, my upper body slowly became debilitated with pain. Initially, I thought it was muscle soreness, but my healthcare professional thought it was trauma from an old car accident. They explained, "Oftentimes, people do not feel the effects of injuries sustained in a car accident until years later." A Chiropractor suggested reducing my weight resistance workouts and taking daily Epsom salt baths. Those recommendations did not help and the pain began to intensify and moved throughout my lower body; then unexplainable, consistent fatigue set in. As time passed, things grew worse and I disclosed again to my healthcare provider who did not have a diagnosis. He dismissed my concerns, saying, "Maybe you're working out too much or struggling with stressful matters." None of these applied to my life at the time, and he did not have another solution.

I knew I was already lifting light-medium weights - it is not like I was training for a fitness competition - yet I accepted his reasoning. Through deductive reasoning, instead of working out three or four days a week, I reduced my regimen to one or two days and began taking over-the-counter pain relief medication as suggested by my physician. However, neither of these options worked after a couple months. Actually, I felt an increase of pain when I decreased my workouts, which was perturbing. The pain decreased once I started to exercise. Generally, I pushed through the pain and stayed active, because I knew that meant some relief for me. With that, I deduced that strenuous activity was not the culprit. I went back to my regular workout regimen and ironically enough, it gave me some relief.

Never in a million years did I think I would look forward to working out especially when I was in pain. Respectively, I sought out various recommendations and suggestions from other healthcare professionals. My research revealed my body pain could be due to high stress, dehydration, lack of nutrients, and even constipation and osteoarthritis. Suggestions included, but not limited to, increase water consumption, reduce stress levels, and increase fiber intake, all of which I did for months on end with no relief.

As time progressed, the pain became more debilitating and my primary physician referred me to a pain specialist. After further evaluation, she gave a shocking diagnosis of Fibromyalgia. Fibromyalgia? I did not believe I had any of the symptoms of Fibromyalgia. The specialist prescribed a popular drug that was newly being tested to treat symptoms of Fibromyalgia and I refused. At the time this drug was mostly used to treat depression and had shown to have many side effects including dizziness and sleepiness, dry mouth, blurred vision, swelling of the hands and feet, and feeling inebriated, to name a few. It did not make sense to me why she would prescribe an antidepressant to treat body pain and fatigue. Neither John, nor I, believed I was depressed. Suffice it to say, I left very discouraged and frustrated when she did not have any suggestions other than pharmaceuticals.

I began using supplements and sought professional counseling to aid with depression and fatigue instead of using pharmaceutical that were recommended. The counselor ruled out depression and it's no surprise the supplements did not improve the symptoms either. I partook in water exercises specializing in body pain. Three months later and still no relief, I sought a second opinion. That physician not only agreed with the initial diagnosis of Fibromyalgia, but also added "early signs" of Lupus, and recommended extending my short-term disability from work. I was elated to take the time off from work, but certainly baffled by the diagnosis. I agreed to extend the work leave, as I thought it would allow me time to investigate and find answers to what was occurring with my body, and of course relieve some of the stress that was brought on by work. I was not convinced of the diagnoses and continued to search for help. By giving me a prescription for an antidepressant, they were telling me loud and clear the bodily pain and exhaustion I endured was all in my head. I was not comfortable with the assessment or the solution.

My Angel

There I was again with a life plagued by illness and no solutions from healthcare professionals or any viable options. I was frustrated and wanted to give up this healthy lifestyle I had spent the last several years developing. I asked myself repeatedly, "What is the point of eating healthy and achieving a balanced lifestyle if I continue to be faced with illnesses?" Once I got rid of the negative thoughts and left my personal pity party, I convinced myself there had to be some solution other than pharmaceutical drugs. Remembering that I had overcome diabetes and was having great success thus far, it gave me the inspiration and determination I needed to move forward. I spent months doing more research, talking with natural healthcare professionals and taking more nutrition and dietary classes. Ultimately, I did discover a few recommendations for slight variation to my diet and supplement use; but it only had a small impact on the symptoms.

I did not have very many pain-free days, but most days I still got out of the house to get moving, with hopes the movement would give me some relief. I frequented local vitamin and herb shops, attended classes and workshops, and started gathering information and putting the puzzle together. The owners or managers of the smaller natural food and vitamin shops were usually available and were willing to share their wealth of knowledge. One day I stumbled upon a vitamin shop in an area I frequented, but never noticed. I caught the tail end of a presentation and the woman mentioned she was an Herbalist. I was somewhat familiar with Herbalists and Naturopaths, but they were not an option for me, because they were not covered by my health insurance. Additionally, at the time, I did not understand enough about the industry to make the sacrifice to pay for "natural health care" out of pocket nor did I grasp there was a difference between supplements and herbs and the benefits. I was curious about this woman's presentation and wanted to find out more about the profession, so afterwards I waited to speak with her. During our conversation, I shared my health concerns and recent diagnosis. Without hesitation, she asked, "Has the doctor checked your vitamin D level?" I responded, "Not that I am aware of." I was intrigued with her compassion and knowledge. She urged me to be tested immediately and I obliged.

The Importance of Vitamin D3

I immediately called my physician to schedule an appointment. During my appointment, I asked for the test and he stated, "It's not something we typically check, but I will do it." He explained that vitamin and mineral levels were not routinely checked without cause because it is not covered by most healthcare plans. I could not comprehend his statement - if vitamins and minerals are essential to the body's function why would it not be checked annually like my cholesterol levels were. There are two main forms of vitamin D: Ergocalciferol (vitamin D2), synthesized by plants (mainly mushrooms and yeast), and Cholecalciferol (vitamin D3) synthesized in the skin when it is exposed to ultraviolet B rays from sunlight. Vitamin D3 is also found in a few food items such as fatty fish. I am aware one way of obtaining vitamin D3 is through sunlight, but I was not aware it shows up in your system as a vitamin.

A level of 20 to 50 nanograms/milliliter is an adequate level to maintain. A level less than 12 ng/ml is indicative of vitamin D deficiency. I was astounded when my results came back a level 3 ng/ml. I was taking a quality multivitamin, eating better and living in sunny Phoenix, Arizona - the valley of sun - for the past several years. How was it possible to be deficient? The physician suggested I immediately begin taking fish oil and over-the-counter vitamin D3 in dosages of at least 5,000 mg per day. The doctor also checked my kidneys to determine if my body was properly absorbing vitamin D, and since they seemed to be functioning properly, there was no other explanation other than I was not taking in enough to support to my system. The manner our bodies receive and absorb vitamin D entail more than living in a sunny climate, and too detailed to explain here. I will share that many say vitamin D deficiency can stem from a lack of sun exposure, a strict vegan diet, or milk allergies. It is recommended for individuals to have an average of 15-20 minutes direct exposure daily to 75% of an uncovered body.

Light at the End of the Tunnel

Within 3-4 months of taking over 5,000 milligrams per day, I noticed positive changes; I was less fatigued and my body pain started to dissipate. I could not believe that I was living in such a debilitating state for almost two years and I could have found relief with a supplement instead of pharmaceuticals. Something that was obvious to an Herbalist, whom I only spent 10 minutes speaking, went undetected by healthcare professionals. During my six-month follow up visit, I reported the positive change to my physician and asked if it was the result of the vitamin D deficiency. He said, "There has been no formal studies conducted, but it has been noted that people with vitamin D deficiency can show signs and symptoms that resemble Fibromyalgia and even Lupus." All I could say to that was "Thank you Lord" for allowing me to listen to that inner voice. A small decision of going into that vitamin shop potentially saved my life. The difference with alternative medicine such as an herbalist is they treat the "whole" person, not put a Band-Aid on the symptoms.

Some new studies suggest that bone pain and muscle weakness can be a symptom of vitamin D deficiency. However, for many people, the symptoms are subtle or can be misdiagnosed. Studies shows that prolong vitamin D deficiency can pose health risks such as cardiovascular disease, cognitive impairment in older adults, severe asthma in children, and certain types of cancer. Research also suggests that vitamin D3 could play a role in the prevention and treatment of a number of different conditions including type 1 and type 2 diabetes, hypertension, glucose intolerance, and multiple sclerosis.

It is not my intent to suggest that body pain, fatigue, Fibromyalgia or Lupus is due to a vitamin D deficiency in everyone. What I am sharing is that healthcare professionals can misdiagnose conditions based on their ignorance about the holistic approach and by only drawing on experience and training from a conventional approach. It is imperative you evaluate the root cause of a problem and look to your body for the answers. In some cases, it may be as simple as taking an herb or supplement or changing your lifestyle habits instead of depending on conventional treatment options. From my involvement with western healthcare practitioners they tend to lean towards prescription medication and surgeries; whereas, alternative healthcare practitioners seek out natural options first. Currently, my level is at a 45 and I no longer take supplements - instead I use herbs and food rich in vitamin D, and the majority of my pain and fatigue are gone. I continue to eat nutritious food and take herbs to efficiently fuel my body and support my daily functions. I did not get the herbalist's information, but wish I could personally thank her for possibly saving my life.

Know Your Vitamin Levels

Consult with a medical or natural healthcare professional before starting any herb or supplement regimen. It is essential to know your vitamin and mineral levels to ensure you are taking the appropriate dosage. Many people think if something is "good" that means more is better. However, this is not always the case. In rare cases, high doses of certain vitamins and minerals in your system can be poisonous and could cause other health problems. More often, if the body receives too much vitamins and minerals at once, most of it is released as waste before it is absorbed. Remember, anything in moderation. The Recommended Dietary Allowances (RDAs) for vitamins on packages shows how much of each vitamin is recommended to be consume each day. However, it's difficult to determine what you need or do not need without knowing your current levels.

- The RDA for vitamins may be used as a guide for each person.
- How much of each vitamin you need depends on your age and gender. Other factors, such as pregnancy, diet, other medication taken and your health, are also important in making a determination.

If you take supplements, DO NOT take more than the RDA unless you know your levels. Be very careful about taking large amounts of fat-soluble vitamin supplements - vitamins A, D, E, and K. These vitamins are stored in fat cells and they can build up in your body and cause harmful effects.

A few of the common supplements, their benefits, and important facts:

- Know the quality of supplements you are putting in your body. In the vitamin/supplement world, most of the time cost does equate better quality. Comparable with food products, you do not want the extra additives or preservatives in your supplements. Many supplements only have a small portion of natural sources and natural does not always mean safe. If you are not familiar with the manufacturer, do a little research; know where it is made, where they are getting the supplies, and if it is non-GMO. You can access any of this information right from your computer or by calling the company.
- Typically, drugstore or supermarket brands may not have the best or highest-quality products. Lesser-quality products may have fillers, additives, preservatives, artificial coloring, and artificial sweeteners. Sadly, you are throwing money away if you are using such products, as they are counterproductive. It is best to purchase your supplements from a health food

- Know what works better for your body and what you can tolerate: tablets, liquid, or powder. Liquid typically absorbs into the bloodstream faster. Talk to your healthcare practitioner.
- Most capsules and gel forms are coated with MSG. There may be health risks associated with high dosage of MSG. Read the package label, asking the vitamin specialist, or research it.
- Have your vitamin/mineral levels tested at your annual wellness check-up. It is possible to have too much or too little of any vitamin or mineral, which could be potentially be harmful.
- According to The National Center for Complementary and Integrative Health, there are many studies and various informational charts available with suggestions on the most important supplement to take daily; such as a complete whole food multivitamin, which includes CoEnzyme Q10, folic acid, and iron.
- Instead of taking a tablet or capsule supplement, it's possible to obtain the majority of all recommended daily vitamins from alfalfa, kelp and dandelion (see Chapter 17).
- Explore high-quality fish oil with both docosahexaenoic acid (DHA) and eicosapentaenoic acid (EPA). Omega-3 fatty acids are essential nutrients that are important in preventing and managing heart disease. It may help to lower blood pressure and increase memory functions.

A few vitamins and minerals that have shown to support your system:

- Alpha lipoic acid has also been known to improve insulin sensitivity.
- Nopal (prickly pear cactus) is known for its anti-inflammatory properties, and can help improve insulin levels.

- Vitamin D3 (which can increase insulin levels in some people), probiotics and chromium (which help improve glucose tolerance by increasing and stabilizing blood sugar levels.), and Magnesium. You decide which is right for your body.
- Vitamin B, vitamin E, magnesium, and zinc, are known to help with fatigues and body pain.
- Psyllium fiber supplement. Eating fiber also helps you feel full, suppresses cravings, promotes digestive health, and helps stabilize blood sugar levels.
- Trace mineral supplements are typically needed due to the lack of quality food that this available.
- Calcium, from herbs and food, for strong bones and overall health. Herbs such as oatstraw, nettle leaf, and chamomile. Food like broccoli, parsnips, sunflower seeds, spinach, kale, figs, avocado.
- Red rice yeast and grapeseed extract can help lower cholesterol.
- Vitamin C is known to boost the immune system and protect against radicals.
- Chlorophyll provides antioxidants, helping to reduce one's mercury level ingested from seafood or environmental factors.

SHOCKING FACT: Typically, vitamin and mineral level tests are not a normal part of the blood panel work during your annual physical. Why is this the case? If it supports the body functions, this should be considered a measure of preventative care. In most cases, I have found that health insurance companies will not cover the entire cost for a complete blood panel work-up. Check with your insurance company about their policy. Until we begin to take a stand as a society, preventative and alternative care will remain our financial responsibility. If we want preventative care, we must take matters into our own hands and take a stand.

CHAPTER 17

Herbs, Teas, and Essential Oils

"Look deep into nature, and then you will understand everything better."

- Albert Einstein

Natural Resources

An herb is a plant or plant part such as leaves, flowers, root, bark or seeds that is used for flavor, scent, and/or potential health-related properties. An herbal supplement may contain a single herb or a mixture of herbs. These may come in forms of extracts, capsule, powder, teas blend, oils, salves, lotion or other substances.

The first known written record of a curative plants was from a Sumerian herbalist from 2200 B.C. Flowers were used for food, protection and to attract love; fragrant plants were worn to heal the body. Egyptians are stated to be the first to use herbs for essential oils and for medicinal, cosmetic, and aromatherapy purposes dating as far back as 1500 B.C. In the 5th century B.C., Greek doctor Hippocrates listed over 400 herbs that were commonly used. Shortly thereafter, countries like China and India were also using various herbs, trees, plants, and flowers as healing methods. Using herbs for medicinal purposes was a way of natural life that continued through the Dark Ages and Renaissance period. Herbs were used on a regular basis and were known to restore, build, maintain and promote health.

Native and indigenous North and South Americans developed their various herbal systems. They learned how to grow and communicate with the plants in order to evoke the plants' medicinal energy, power and healing agents. As these traditions evolved, they were passed down to other generations by word of mouth. Many of these methods and traditions were lost as cultures were destroyed in South and North America, as well as Europe, in the early 1500s. Ambitious people, through research and talking with "old school" master teachers, rediscovered invaluable ancient teachings. Research has shown that use of herbs can be beneficial to radiant health and well-being, whereas many other supplements only provide artificial fillers and toxins. Scientists have found that folic acid prevents certain birth defects and can be found in herbs such as nettle leaf and oatstraw. Nettle leaf and oatstraw are loaded with calcium, vitamin E and a lot of minerals; whereas other popular herbs such as Echinacea are traditionally used to improve and support the immune system. Other herbs include: Ginkgo biloba - improves memory; flaxseed - lowers cholesterol; lavender - to relax; and the list of remedies goes on. See more at the end of this chapter.

Know Your History

The history of essential oils is intertwined with the history of herbal medicine, which has been an integral part of Eastern medicine practices for many centuries. Herbal medicine has been used for more than treating minor ailments and disease; it has been instrumental in providing life-enhancing benefits. In most ancient cultures, people believed plants to be magical, and for thousands of years herbs were used as much for ritual purposes as they were for medicine and food. According to many medicinal herbalist and healers, Greek philosopher Aristotle believed that plants had psyches. They used aromatic plants to make oils, ointments, and incense; these were elements of religious and therapeutic practices in early cultures worldwide. Frankincense and myrrh, known as the perfume of the gods, are two such examples. Burning incense and sage for spiritual rituals is another; it was believed that it provided a connection between the physical and spiritual worlds, a link between the mundane and the Divine.

Healing with herbal plants, sometimes referred to as botanical, is not a new revelation. Both humans and animals sought healing from the natural resources available to them, in barks, seeds, berries, roots, fruit bodies, and other parts of the plants. Awareness of medicinal plants usage is a result of the many years of struggles against illnesses and finding a "cure" for health problems. Hippocrates used many herbal remedies in his practice and wrote the famous words "Let foods be thy medicines, and medicines thy food." He wrote about the medicinal properties of willow bark and how it could be used for fevers and pain.

Although pharmacies could be found in many places dating back to 750, it was not until the 1700's, that scientists began synthesizing active compounds from plant parts (herbs) such as the willow bark to make aspirin. Yet, modern pharmaceutical drugs really did not begin to displace natural remedies until the 20th century. Due to supply and demand, modern science and the pharmaceutical industry imposed contemporary technology by creating synthetic supplements and drugs to emulate the healing effects of medicinal plants and herbs. This was demonstrated with the introduction of insulin injections to manage diabetes in the 1920s. Shortly after, people's belief and opinion of herbs began to change, yet many herbalists continued to practice. The formation of the Council on Medical Education (CME) by the American Medical Association (AMA) in 1904 established standards for medical practices, which forced many herbalists to cease using herbs for medicinal purposes.

When the medical education system became standardized, they imposed strict operational processes on herbal teachings and practices, some of which are still in existence today. Between 1910 and 1935, these changes affected many schools offering training in homeopathy, naturopathy, and chiropractic training, causing more than half of these schools to either merge with larger universities or close down. It was not until 1937 that medicinal herbs were re-introduced in North American. Of course, there are usually good reasons to regulate and raise the standards of educational institutions; there is also something to be said for supporting different methods and alternative treatments. The medical system is beginning to slowly change and accept alternative schools of medicine including Osteopathic Schools (DO-Doctor of Osteopathic Medicine); for-profit and non-profit accredited schools are offering herbalism and alternative medicine in their curricula. It is my hope that due to the increasing awareness of potential side effects of some supplements and drugs, the usage of natural herbs will continue to increase in popularity.

Herbs Have Healing Effects

Some herbs can have drug like effects, and few can be strong enough to cause health risks. Therefore, they should be used with caution and with professional assistance, especially if you are using pharmaceuticals. The difference between supplements, pharmaceuticals and herbs, is that herbs are without added chemical or toxins that could cause potential harm to the body. There is a long history of documented benefits of using herbs. When used over time as a preventative measure, they have significant rewards including longevity. Usage is easily regulated, and any particular plant or herb can be used for multiple conditions. Medicinal plants and herbs have been recorded as a healing agent for diabetes, cancer, heart disease, digestive disorders, respiratory problems, and skin conditions. Herbal medicine has come full circle, with the increase of natural health and wellness, with improvements in analysis, advances in clinical research, and better quality control; it is also becoming more valuable in mainstream treatment and disease prevention. Additionally, it is more cost effective and has fewer side effects than other conventional treatment methods.

As a young girl, I do not recall going to the doctor for anything other than major incidents that required stitches or urgent care. It was common for my grandparents or mother to use elixirs to heal ailments and for preventative care. I recall drinking Senna tea on a Saturday evening, at least once a month. It was used to clean the blood and colon of impurities. Senna Leaf (Senna pod) is commonly used to alleviate constipation, stimulate the colon, improve digestion, and relieve heartburn and gas. Although Senna has many healing properties, when used long term, it served to a disadvantage. Unbeknownst to my parents, long term use of Senna can cause laxative dependence. Using herbs was passed down through many generations in my family; they knew of the many benefits but not the side effects, as was the case with Senna. Most herbs are safe for regular and long-term use but few must be used with caution. As I grew older, it was easy for me to accept herbs as a natural way of life, due to my upbringing. After research, education and personal experience, I became more convinced that herbal remedies were the best alternative to conventional resources for me and my family.

Asthma Strikes

I recall being in a frantic state when my daughter was diagnosed with asthma at six months old. My mother put her "naturopathic, ole West Indian school" hat on and used her knowledge of essential oils and herbs to restore her lungs. She did not agree with the western medicine approach of treatment and urged me not to put my daughter on a breathing machine nor the inhaler. My mother successfully raised seven children and she shared that one of my brothers had asthma as a child in which she treated with herbs. Thanks to the treatments my mother used, my daughter did not take the inhaler and was not put on an asthma machine. During the herbal treatment period, we made routine visits to her healthcare specialist to monitor her progress - the doctor could not believe that she showed no signs of a lung infection, breathing difficulty or other asthmatic symptoms after a year.

My daughter is now in her mid-20s, and has not had any problems with her lungs. She was never restricted from any physical activities; she participated in many physically challenging sports, including three years of running competitive track and even today, she continues to enjoy running as a form of physical activity. Thanks to my mother's knowledge of herbs, my daughter continues to have fully developed and functional lungs. This is just one of many scenarios of how my mother used food, herbs, plants, essential oils, and other natural means to prevent or treat bruises, ear infections, fractures, headache, cold/flu, stomach pain, and fevers with her children and grandchildren. Herbal remedies have been informally practiced throughout many generations in my family and will hopefully continue since my daughter, along with her cousins, have benefited from it all of their lives and they understand the purpose and use of herbs.

The Miracle of Essential Oils and Teas

In the late 1700s as the pharmaceutical industry grew, herbal traditions began to fade throughout the world. People became superstitious and looked for a quick recovery from synthetic drugs; this, combined with ignorance and embellished rituals, deemed these plants less effective. As master teachers of alternative medicine resurface and teachings are being reintroduced, many individuals are returning to herbs for their healing and therapeutic properties. Countless essential oils, herbs and teas are now used worldwide for medicinal and aromatherapy purposes.

A few of the most common herbs and their benefits (not limited to what's listed), some important facts, and their common use are listed below. However, check with your healthcare practitioner before starting any new practices.

Essential Oils

- Lavender oil - Used for relaxation and stress relief. Mix it with aloe vera to relieve sunburn, bug bites, and poison ivy rashes.
- Eucalyptus oil - Helps with reducing fever and relieving pain.
- Geranium oil - Mixed with the above two oils together in a diffuser for relaxation or allergy/sinus.
- Tea tree oil - Helps treat cuts, bruises/scrapes; it's a healing agent.
- Rosemary oil - Use with peppermint and ginger root to help heal sprains.
- Peppermint oil or leaves - Relieves headaches (gently massage into the temples); great for digestive concerns.
- Black seed oil or oil of oregano can be used as an antibiotic or to boost immune system.
- Frankincense and myrrh oil - An excellent immunity and inflammatory healer.

Caution: Dilute essential oils before applying to the skin, especially on children; they are better used in a diffuser. If you ingest, make certain it can be taken orally.

Herbs

Herbs, plants, flowers, or barks: Many of these herbs are used in combination for greater effects and benefits. They can be taken orally as a tea blend - steeping in hot water allows the healing properties to be drawn out. Herbal recipes are passed down through generations of master teachers to help with blood circulation, blood sugar levels, hair, nails and skin, liver detox, balancing the hormonal and female reproduction system, and strengthening the male prostate, among many others. These are not to be used as recreational tea but for medicinal purposes under the advisement of an Herbalist. As a trained Herbalist, I have the privilege of having access to many of these formulas, which I personally hand blend for my clients. You can find these on my website, www.gailparkerlifestyle.com

The healing properties or constituents of an herb can also be drawn out through the process of making elixir, extract, salve, cream, oil or lotion. In addition, herbs have been traditionally used in cooking recipes and nutritious purposes.

- Pine bark extract - Suggested 30-100 mg daily for perimenopausal and menopause issues.
- Oregano - Helps the digestive and immune system.
- Fenugreek - Helps new mothers with lactation production.
- Lemon grass or slippery elm bark - For digestive and stomach concerns.
- Cleavers and Echinacea - Strengthens the Lymph System.
- Chamomile - Used for calcium, iron, magnesium, manganese, and vitamin A.
- Echinacea, Red Clover, and Astragalus - Aids in boosting the immune system.
- Isabgol - 1 tbsp. in water before bed to help with constipation and cleansing of the colon.
- Passionflower, St. John's Wort, Lemon Balm or Mother's Wort - Used to calm anxiety, depression, and IBS. These groups of herbs also help ease the nervous system.

The three herbs listed below contain a potency of vitamins and minerals. Their constituents make an excellent nutritious blend for multivitamin. They include but are not limited to:

- Dandelion - Strengthens and cleanses the liver, gallbladder and kidneys. Used to reduce blood pressure.
- Kelp - Contains Iodine, Calcium, Iron, Sodium, Potassium, Phosphorus, Magnesium, Protein, Carotene, Riboflavin, vitamin A, B1, B3, B5, B6, B9, B12, C, E and Zinc.

- Alfalfa - Amino Acids, digestive enzymes, vitamins A, C D, E, B and K, Calcium, Phosphorous, Magnesium, Iron, Potassium, and trace minerals.

Tea

"There doesn't seem to be a downside to tea," says American Dietetic Association representative Katherine Tallmadge, MA, RD, LD. "I think it's a great alternative to coffee drinking. First, tea has less caffeine. It's pretty well established that the compounds in tea - their flavonoids - are good for the heart and may reduce cancer."

For centuries, various parts of the plant have been used for medicinal teas, whereas, with recreational teas, only the leaves are used. The plant leaves vary in caffeine grade from zero to high. Many of the tea leaves below can be combined with any of the herbs listed above into formulas creating an herbal blends for recreational or medicinal purposes.

- **White tea** is the least processed of all teas, which is valued for its mild delicate flavor. It is known as the "Emperor's drink," and was reserved for royalty going back as far as the Tang Dynasty. White tea is made from the same plant as green, black, and yellow tea (Camellia sinensis), which means it shares many of green tea's wonderful health benefits, including reducing cholesterol, decreasing blood pressure, and lowering the risk of heart disease. Unlike green tea, it is produced from the unopened buds of a tea plant, which is uncured and unfermented. This is what gives white tea its characteristic clean "white" or "silver" appearance. White tea does not require panning, rolling, or shaking, but must be carefully picked at the right time to yield the highest quality of tea.
- **Rooibos tea** ("red" or "herbal") surprisingly is not from a tea tree or flower. It is actually derived from a broom-shaped legume that grows in the fertile lands of South Africa.

Traditionally, local people would scale high mountains to harvest the leaves of the rooibos plant. As a naturally caffeine-free tea, rooibos has been shown to aid in digestion, alleviate nervous tension, relieve allergies, and allow the body to retain iron (as opposed to losing it through waste fluids). Rooibos tea can be used to satiate sugar cravings, especially at night, due to its naturally sweet taste. Rooibos can be blended easily with many fruits and spices, and is especially complimented when blended with natural vanilla.

- **Green tea** originated in China and quickly spread throughout Asia; in recent years it has also become popular in North America. Many say it has an energizing, yet relaxing effect on the body. Green tea has been praised by numerous medical and scientific studies for its health benefits, which may include: reducing cholesterol, lowering the risk of heart disease, lowering blood pressure, improving the skin, elevating mood, protecting brain cells and aiding weight loss. In addition, green tea has a great anti-inflammatory property and is loaded with cancer-fighting antioxidants. Green tea is packed with catechins, which are powerful antioxidants that repair and protect the body's cells. The best way to drink it is in lukewarm water, as the use of boiling water destroys the catechins. When adding lemon to green tea, it increases the vitamin C, making catechins easier to absorb. Although there are many benefits, green tea is caffeinated and, therefore, can have a negative effect on blood sugar levels.

It is very popular to find green tea extract in everything from bottled beverages and dietary supplements to cosmetics. But the quality or amount of tea in many of these products has not been recorded or shown to have the same benefits as using natural tea leaves.

- **Black tea** is more oxidized than green tea, generally giving it a stronger, more complex flavor and caffeinated kick. Black tea gets its name from the color of the oxidized leaves and can vary in strength and taste according to the characteristics and region where it was grown. It is by far the most popular type of tea in North America. Unlike green tea, which has a shorter shelf life, black tea will retain its flavor for over a year. Black teas are often named for the regions where they are produced; it is so valuable to the cultures that produce them, that they drink it regularly. Black tea was even used as a form of currency in parts of Mongolia, Tibet, and Siberia in the 18th and early 19th centuries.

A few other teas such as oolong, chia, and Pu-erh are considered a black tea. Many processed teas and tea bags sold in grocery stores may not have the same effects and benefits as herbal or pure tea leaves from an herbal specialty vendor. The same protocol should be used here as with vitamin; all teas or herbal tea blends are not created equal. Therefore, the effects and benefits will vary accordingly. In order to get the best quality teas, purchase them from a specialty tea or herb vendor/store that sells in bulk.

Any herbs, plants, flowers, barks, roots, and teas leaves can be combined in tinctures or compounds for various healing benefits. Before you start usage of any essential oils or herbs, make sure you speak with an experienced natural healthcare professional.

SHOCKING FACT: Recently, the World Health Organization estimated that 80% of people worldwide rely on herbal medicines for some part of their primary health care. In Germany, about 600-700 plant-based medicines are available and are prescribed by some 70% of German physicians. In the past 20 years in the United States, public dissatisfaction with the cost of prescription medications, combined with an interest in returning to natural or organic remedies, has led to an increase in herbal medicine use.

CHAPTER 18

"Food As Thy Medicine"

"We all eat, and it would be a sad waste of opportunity to eat badly."

- Anna Thomas

Superfoods

The best way to get the recommended amount of daily vitamins is to eat a balanced diet that contains a wide variety of fruits, vegetables, legumes (dried beans), lentils, and whole grains. Many of these are considered "superfoods" - nature's vitamins and mineral supplements. Superfoods are commonly known as whole foods naturally concentrated with essential nutrients. A dietary supplement is just that - a supplement - and not the primary means of providing the nutrients the body requires. Superfoods provide the whole spectrum of nutrients that only nature can provide. Due to the lack of nutrients in our food today and what is available to the public, whole food and herbal supplements can be a crucial aspect of your daily regimen. There are factors that prohibit us from getting the daily allowance from food, including limited access to certain food, the quality of the food available, the quantity needed to ingest, and ensuring regular usage. Most people have found it more convenient to take a high quality whole food vitamin or herb until such time that you can obtain the daily allowance from natural food sources.

"One cannot think well, love well, and sleep well, if one has not dined well." - Virginia Woolf

Mary's Health Concerns

At 76 years old Mary came to me because of her failing health. She could not figure out what was going wrong and had recently weathered several health issues despite being on prescription medication to prevent the very concerns that occurred. Her health concerns included blocked arteries, high cholesterol, and a brush with diabetes. She shared that in her younger years she exercised regularly and was embarrassed to say that it was more for vanity - how she looked, rather than how she felt, was more important to her at that time. She has some "old school" knowledge about herbs and natural remedies, but did not practice them consistently.

She was caught up the vain world that traps many of us, and she focused on what she looked like on the outside, instead of focusing on her inner health. When her exterior (physical appearance) showed little changes despite activities, she, like so many of us, gave up working out and did not see the point. She thought, "It's an age factor and there is nothing I can do so why bother exercising?" She did not make the connection that exercise aids in weight loss, and has tremendous benefits for muscle strength, healthy bones, brain activity, and mental health; however, weight loss is primarily due to dietary habits.

As she decreased her physical activity and continued unhealthy eating habits, her health began to decline. As a result, instead of refining her eating habits and using herbs and supplements, she believed the prognosis, diagnosis, and recommendations given to her by healthcare professionals, without ever researching or questioning the information. At times, she was given pharmaceuticals to prevent certain diseases and ailments when she did not have any symptoms; for example, she was prescribed high blood pressure medications, although her blood pressure was within a normal range. The reason they prescribed it was due to her age and for preventive measures. Whatever happened to natural prevention measures, first? Mary believed if she followed their recommendations she would not be sick. When heart problems, high cholesterol, and high blood pressure struck, she could not understand why since she was taking prescription medication *as preventative measures. Most recently, it was discovered that the medication Mary was given several years prior is now being linked to causing diabetes in many individuals. Mary has a strong predisposition for diabetes in her family history and recently she was put on medication to regulate her blood sugar levels. Her indulgence also could have attributed to the damage - things such as the overuse of white sugar, artificial sweeteners, diet soda, cookies, pastries, candy and dairy.*

Once she had a better understanding of how to use food and herbs to aid her health, she began to see improvements while still on the medication. Fortunately, she now has a healthcare professional who listened to her concerns, is knowledgeable in natural therapy and respects her working with a natural healthcare provider to eventually discontinue the use of prescription medications. He agreed with her incorporating alternative methods, and agreed to monitor her while decreasing the dosage, or discontinuing some of her medication when possible. The great thing is that with patience and time, she is making great strides. Mary is now well aware of the importance of not just physical activity but eating healthy, reducing stress and using herbs and supplements to achieve radiant health.

The Future of Medicine

I have had a few negative experiences with conventional healthcare providers throughout the years. If you are one who has been lucky enough to have a healthcare professional who supports alternative health care and uses medication only as a last resort and short term, I applaud that person. I do believe that some prescription medications do have its place in aiding diseases, but should only be used short term in an emergency and as a last resort.

Keep in mind, all herbs, vitamins, supplements and essential oils are NOT created equal. Often times, chiropractors and other natural healthcare practitioners either carry or can order a high-quality product or professional strength if you are not satisfied with what you find at a local natural or herbal store. I urge you to research any supplements that are lab created.

It is vital to make every attempt to obtain most nutrients from your food and herbs. Therefore, it is critical to eat fruits, vegetables, beans/lentils, spices, plants, roots, and whole grains. Not regularly eating a sufficient amount of these food groups may increase the risk for health problems, including heart disease, cancer, and poor bones (osteoporosis). Remember, it is necessary to speak with a medical or natural healthcare professional before adding any supplement regimen to your lifestyle.

A few of the common food sources, their benefits, and important facts:

- Apple cider vinegar, baking soda, lemon, and lime, have been known to aid with the digestive system, acid reflux, stabilizing BSL (blood sugar level) and decreasing the body's acidity while increasing alkalinity.
- Bananas and berries have many benefits, including pectin, which stabilizes blood sugar and gives you energy. Recall these are simple carbs - identify where they fall on the glycemic index chart for your individual needs.
- Apples, pears, beans, and berries contain dietary fiber, which promote a healthy colon. They are rich in antioxidants and flavonoids. The phytonutrients and antioxidants in apples and berries may help reduce the risk of developing cancer, hypertension, diabetes, and heart disease.
- Coconut is a good source for fatty acids and fiber.
- Pumpkin seeds contain zinc, which promotes a healthy immune system.
- Turmeric Root (Curcumin) - Turmeric is an herb that gives curry its yellow color. Curcumin is the main active ingredient in turmeric. In order to get the full benefits of turmeric, use the actual root not curcumin or turmeric extract. It has powerful anti-inflammatory effects and is a very strong antioxidant. It also improves brain function, and possibly

helps to prevent and treat certain types of cancer, Alzheimer's, and depression, among many others.
- Ginger Root (not the candy form) is great as an anti-inflammatory with arthritis and osteoarthritis; it helps with morning sickness or nausea, reduces heart disease risk, muscle pain and soreness, stabilizes blood sugar levels, and relieves indigestion, menstrual cramps and many other benefits.
- Cayenne pepper and cacao powder promote antioxidants and anti-inflammatory.
- Cucumber is great for hydrating and fighting inflammation.
- Broccoli and cabbage contain calcium, which helps build strong bones and improves overall health.
- Parsley and cilantro are great for natural internal cleansing and chelation.
- Chia seeds contain fiber, protein, fat, calcium, magnesium and much more.
- Aloe Vera gel or juice helps regulate blood sugar, aids the digestive system, and cleanses the colon.
- Flaxseeds help lower blood pressure, cardiovascular disease, hot flashes, and cleanses the colon
- Guava contains soluble fiber, vitamin C, and potassium.
- Legumes are a good source of fiber. It helps improve liver function and blood sugar.

FAT-SOLUBLE VITAMINS

Fat-soluble vitamins, including multivitamins, come from a variety of foods:

Vitamin A:
- Dark-colored fruit
- Dark leafy vegetables
- Eggs
- Liver, beef, and fish

Vitamin D:
- Fish (fatty fish such as salmon, sardines, mackerel, herring, tuna and orange roughy)
- Cod liver oil
- Green leafy vegetables (kale, spinach, and collard)
- Beef liver

Vitamin E:
- Avocado
- Dark green vegetables (spinach, broccoli, asparagus, turnip greens)
- Oils (safflower, palm, and sunflower)
- Papaya and mango
- Seeds and nuts (almonds, sunflower)
- Sweet Potato, butternut squash

Vitamin K:
- Cabbage
- Cauliflower
- Fortified whole grain cereals
- Dark green vegetables (broccoli, Brussels sprouts, asparagus)
- Dark leafy vegetables (spinach, kale, collards, turnip greens)
- Fish, liver, beef, eggs

WATER-SOLUBLE VITAMINS:

Water-soluble vitamins (found in multivitamin) come from a variety of foods:

Biotin:
- Chocolate
- Egg yolk (most beneficial when the whole egg is eaten)
- Legumes
- Nuts

- Organ meats (liver, kidney)
- Brewer's yeast (avoid if you have sinus problems or a lot of inflammation)

Folate:

- Asparagus and broccoli
- Beets
- Brewer's yeast
- Dried beans (soaked and cooked pinto, navy, and kidney, and lima)
- Fortified whole grain cereals (milling and processing removes a lot of this vitamin from most cereals)
- Green, leafy vegetables (spinach and romaine lettuce)
- Lentils
- Oranges or fresh squeezed orange juice

Niacin (vitamin B3):

- Avocado
- Eggs
- Enriched sprouted breads and fortified whole grain cereals
- Fish (tuna and saltwater fish)
- Lean meats
- Legumes
- Nuts
- Red Potato
- Poultry

Pantothenic acid:

- Avocado
- Broccoli, kale, and other vegetables in the cabbage family
- Eggs
- Legumes and lentils

- Mushrooms
- Organ meats (liver and kidney)
- Poultry
- Sweet potatoes
- Fortified whole-grain cereals

Thiamine (vitamin B1):

- Egg
- Lean red meats
- Legumes and beans
- Nuts and seeds
- Organ meats (liver and kidney)
- Peas

Pyroxidine (vitamin B6):

- Avocado
- Banana
- Legumes (dried beans)
- Meat
- Nuts
- Poultry
- Fortified whole grains

Vitamin B12:

- Meat
- Eggs
- Organ meats (liver and kidney)
- Poultry
- Shellfish

SHOCKING FACT: According to "Science Based Medicine," eating is an intrinsic and essential part of what we do and who we are.

The idea that the body can rebel violently to everyday foods can be difficult to believe, but it is real, and the number of such cases is growing rapidly. For example, allergies are a result of a weakened immune system and inflammation with multiple biochemical pathways triggered in response to a specific antigen. "Allergy" can be described as a mild skin reaction or respiratory distress, right through to bigger, life-threatening reactions. Healthcare professionals agree that the majority of food-related allergic reactions are not life threatening; rather, they are silent allergies. However, they can wreak havoc on the system, silently affecting how you process and digest your food and triggering the release of toxins - without you even noticing it.

Knowing your allergies is a large component of a healthy bodily process. If the digestive system is not well managed, it can lead to problems like colon spasms and constipation, with the latter of these problems capable of creating a buildup of toxins and inflammation in the body that in turn triggers greater health issues. You may want to consider getting an allergy test done by a natural healthcare practitioner in order to assist in this process. Natural healthcare practitioners suggest having an allergy test done via blood sample at least every 5-10 years as preventive care. As the body ages, things change internally and that means hormonal and body chemistry changes resulting in allergies.

FINAL WORDS

"Wholesome foods are the way to go for optimal health. Blaming disease on one aspect of our diet is foolish and unrealistic." - Author Unknown

Through my 20 plus years, (and counting) I have been living successfully with diabetes without the use of medication. Throughout this journey, I have discovered the secret to my success is creating an intentional lifestyle which includes regular mental cleansing, stress management, making smart food choices, meal planning, staying active and moderate use of supplements and herbs. I have found it is nearly impossible to achieve maximum results unless I have incorporated all the components; they are each a part of the health and wellness puzzle and must work hand-in-hand. I know firsthand, because I have tried several times without incorporating all facets simultaneously and time after time, I did not obtain maximum results. Many of you have probably tried your own version only to wonder why things have not changed.

Further, because of these changes, I regularly receive compliments on my healthy physical appearance. Although flattering, what is more important to me is that I feel amazing on the inside. Knowing that I have reversed diabetes, overcome weight issues, acid reflux, constipation/IBS, sinus, fibromyalgia, severe acne, rosacea and alopecia is an enormous and gratifying accomplishment. This is not a one size fits all approach; I suggest you take these principles and systems and tailor them to suit your lifestyle, challenges and goals. These secrets should continue to act as your foundation to health and wellness, even as you age. I often make the analogy between the body and a car. With age, cars suffer wear and tear, and as parts start to falter, we must repair them accordingly; using the principles given here can help your body run optimally and prevent unnecessary damage. I have made it this far without any further use of conventional treatments. I continue to stay positive and treat my body as God's temple, giving it only the best care.

Now it's time for you to also take responsibility for your weight loss, migraine, acne, sleepless nights, joint and back pain, constipation, arthritis, high blood pressure, high cholesterol, digestive problems, hormonal, diabetes, or any other health concern. Big or small, it is time to take back control and regain a radiant well-being. I urge you to discover what motivates you to better health and to limit future health concerns. Do not wait until the engine blows out on your car before you realize you should have changed the oil. Likewise, do not wait until you start to feel pain and nervous system failure before implementing these principles. It is so much easier to take preventative measures than being reactive trying to undo a serious condition. Your motivation should not solely focus on losing weight or getting down to a certain size; let's face it, our external shell will change as we age, and as humans, we are rarely content with our physical appearance. You can, however, be feel better with knowing that you do not suffer from obesity and other major health issues. You are sleeping better at night, have utilization of all limbs, and have a better chance of preventing a heart attack or going blind, all because you took matters into your own hands and accepted responsibility for our health. There is an old Chinese saying, *"The time to start digging a well is before you feel thirsty."* Similarly, the time to start attending to your health is before you become sick.

It is troubling to me when people say, "I wish I could look like you or be your size." My response is, "With all due respect, no you don't." First, you should want to look like *you*. Additionally, it may not be biologically possible to be my size because of different genetic stature, but you *can* be healthy and look amazing according to your body type and genetic makeup. Are you prepared to make the necessary changes and commitment toward achieving your ultimate lifestyle? It takes work, and if you are willing to change your mindset, get rid of the excuses, and make better choices, you can look and feel healthier and extend your life expectancy. Obtaining my current health and physique took years of commitment, trial and error; research, attending workshops, making sacrifices and self-discipline. I am not perfect and I do falter, but what I have learned is to remain steadfast and not become discouraged. Whatever you do, do not create unnecessary frustration and unrealistic goals by comparing yourself to others. If you must compete, compete with yourself; set small attainable goals and build upon them.

Some say it is all in the genes. I believe that is a fallacy, as I would have been destined to die at an early age from obesity, diabetes, and heart problems, like many of my family members. Overcoming my genetic predisposition for diabetes and other health concerns is my motivation to continue on this journey and to be better with every passing day. My mindset change and determination allowed me to overcome sickness and say, "Yes" to feeling and looking better. I did not want to suffer amputation, blindness, or other physical problems. I believe it is within my control, and I am willing to put forth the effort to change my destiny. I now have such a strong foundation and confidence level about my health from all the things I have learned, and it is that confidence that keeps me going on days that I become frustrated and want to give up.

I could easily attribute my poor health to conventional practices and processed food, but I would still be sick. Shifting the responsibility to external factors and taking it off of me solves nothing; we must accept a certain level of responsibility for what happens to us. Our negative experiences generally keep us stagnant and cause us to continue our negative behaviors. We inflict pain upon ourselves by our actions: eating *comfort food*, being too busy to take care of ourselves, and constantly putting others before ourselves. It is time to take care of you! Many of us have emotional baggage, but it is a matter of how we allow it to affect our lives, here and now. *"It has been said that time heals all wounds. I do not agree. The wounds remain. Time - the mind, protecting its sanity - covers them with some scar tissue and the pain lessens, but it is never gone,"* - Rose Kennedy. If you are not happy with your body, life, or health, there is only one person who can do something about it: YOU!

Here are some important tips to help you move forward:

- Set small manageable, attainable, and realistic goals and keep building upon them. Refrain from becoming stagnant and complacent.
- This lifestyle change takes time, so be patient; it is a marathon not a sprint. We now live in a very fast paced world and we expect instant results and gratification. Permanent change takes time, just as a good 25-year scotch takes time to mature. Be patient with yourself, the results will happen.
- Show mental tough love toward yourself; do not give into every unhealthy craving or eat everything that is placed before you. It is okay to treat yourself, but do not allow your *treats* to be your motivation or reward for wellness. For example, do not say, *if I work out three times this week, I can have a latte or buy shoes*. Let's be real, if you want that latte or those shoes, you will get it regardless. Dare to be different!
- Keep a written journal or use a mobile app - track how you feel and what you eat. You will not know what to do unless you know what you have done or how it is working. Through this process, you may undergo a lot of mental and physical changes, it is important to know where you have been (what you have accomplished) to know where you are going (to determine your successes). Become very in tuned with your body.

- Find a support group, a natural healthcare provider, health coach, or a friend to hold you accountable.
- Refrain from following any one particular diet, boxing yourself into one category or putting labels on yourself - this is a lifestyle which allows for flexibility and individuality. When you can freely make adjustments along the way where needed, it creates a better chance of success.
- Hold yourself responsible and accountable for all your actions. Remember, you always have a choice. Choose right!
- Get in the habit of planning and preparing weekly meals and snacks. This can prevent binge eating, going hungry, and eating unhealthy foods.
- Whether on the road, at an event, a restaurant, or a friend's house, have a plan when eating away from home. I normally eat a light meal before going to an event if I am not familiar with of the menu. This prevents me from making unhealthy choices or starving myself.
- Refrain from or limit eating fast food or at restaurants. When eating out at a restaurant, request to have your meal prepared according to your liking - even if it's not on the menu. Choose to have meat grilled, baked, sautéed in a little olive oil or broiled; avoid fried foods. Request for vegetables to be steamed or sautéed using very little olive oil; ask that less salt to be applied. Instead of bacon or ham, ask for applesauce, salad or seasonal fruit.
- If you must eat fried food, it is best to eat it in moderation and occasionally. If frying at home use oil appropriate for high temperature i.e. sesame, avocado, or palm oil and never reuse the same oil.
- Know which oils are best for cooking variations: sautéing - many oils are great, including avocado, coconut, grapeseed, olive, sesame and high oleic safflower and sunflower oils; for baking - coconut, palm, and high oleic safflower and sunflower oil work best.

- Avoid use of butter, vegetable or canola oil. If you must use butter, use grass fed and unsalted.
- It is important to reward yourself with responsible options such as fresh fruit sorbet or dark chocolate. Make your own desserts i.e. brownies, cupcakes, pumpkin pie, and dairy-free ice cream and eat in moderation.
- Stress is sometimes unavoidable but it can be manageable; deal with it quickly and appropriately when it happens.
- Worrying is an intentional behavior. Studies show the things most people worry about never happen. Bobby McFerrin's popular song, "Don't Worry, Be happy", is a motto to live by.
- Turn off the negative chatter and turn on the positive thoughts.
- Be aware of the naysayers, even if they come disguised as a friend, mother, sister, spouse, or significant other. Just because you want to change does not mean they do or will be supportive of your goals. You may have to temporarily limit your contact with certain people and/or change your environment.

Keys to Success

Making better choices means taking responsibility for yours and your family's life and health. Maintaining better health is more than just eating well and taking supplements; it must include managing stress, meditation, quality of sleep, being physically active and prioritizing you. Prioritizing you does not mean everyone else suffers. It means making time to take care of your well-being first. Change your perception and begin living the way you want – not the way you used to.

A balanced lifestyle is valuable. I encourage you to start this program with a positive mindset. Do not believe for one minute that I am some health food guru. I do not live a "perfect" life, and I am not striving to be the "perfect" healthy person; I want to be and feel at my best, prevent illness and disease, and live a radiant lifestyle. I believe in eating most of what I desire within moderation and without doing harm to my body i.e. eating ice cream once or twice a year. Over time, your taste buds will change and the cravings for unhealthy foods will soon diminish.

A balanced lifestyle includes having stressful moments, but over time you will master how to quickly let go of the worry, fear, and stress, and not allow it to linger causing harm. I have armed myself with techniques to better deal with life matters. I have practiced talking about solutions, not problems. I have changed my perspective to look at the glass as half full. I do encounter bad days when I don't feel like engaging in physical activity and ordinarily I push through, while on rare occasions, I listen to my body and do not force a half-hearted attempt. This is permitted as long as you do not allow old habits to permanently return and stand between you and your goals.

Throughout your journey you will encounter frustration and have weak moments; it is normal to have such thoughts and feelings. Focus on the solution and the goal, not the problem. Do not give up when things do not go quite as planned; put it in the past and keep looking forward to a fresh start. When we continuously look back to the past, it is like putting a car in drive while focusing on the rear view mirror - the results are usually not favorable. Do not debate the power of a successful mindset. You have a choice; make the decision to start now, right where you are, in this moment. Furthermore, one sure way to *get different results is by doing something different.* Many of you may want to improve your current wellness status, but do not want to try anything different to achieve it. You have to do something different to get different results.

You cannot change the laws of physics; what you put in, is what you get out. Your body is going to change; thus, you have to determine what that change will look like and how you want to live in it while it is happening. Indeed, many of my clients are afraid that if they start the process, they will fail, or they are simply afraid of the unknown. Remember: *"You only fail when you don't try."*

Learn from mistakes and you should never have to repeat them. If you do not try and fail, how do you ever grow or have successes to celebrate? You have to take a risk and make changes, because the risk of death is greater than taking a risk to accomplish better health. Someone once told me, "It's in doing that you discover," and I found this to be very true. You must start venturing out, exploring, researching, and reading; this is the "doing" component. Once you begin to take those first steps, you will have broadened your horizon, expanded your knowledge and you can then implement a plan; this is the "discovering" aspect. It's the law of the universe - start to seek out and you shall find. I began my journey to find a better way to live healthy without using medication. I did not know where to start. All I knew was that I wanted options that would take me in the direction of extending my life. That is how I discovered the information I am sharing with you. Therefore, I am asking you to trust the process even when it does not make sense to you.

"Everything in your life is a reflection of what you feel you deserve." - Author Unknown.

I encourage you to take it day-by-day and stand strong in your journey. You are on the road to living well and feeling better. Personally, when I accepted that "I did not know what I did not know" and forgave myself of my unintentional, but harmful past behaviors, I opened up for growth and improvement. I wanted to feel on the inside what everyone saw on the outside. I realized it was realistic to live without getting headaches, feeling nauseous, consistent dry mouth and thirst, passing out, and shakiness, just by changing how and what I ate and treated my body. After over 20 years on this road to defy diabetes and other health concerns, I can honestly say I am as healthy on the inside as it reflects on the outside.

To live a healthier lifestyle, we must then accept our society, as it is, but advocate for change and adapt accordingly. Ideally, most of us would love to have our own garden or shop regularly at a farmer's market, and make all of our food from scratch. In reality, we live far from our food sources, buy foods with extended shelf life, and barely have time to eat dinner, much less prepare it. We must incorporate methods to bring balance, slow down and prioritize in order to live the healthiest life possible. Most people think they cannot eat healthy on a budget or cannot do anything about the food in the grocery store, but such thinking is limited. Actually, you should be eating better with a limited income. You should not have money to buy the "crap" foods, if you prioritize purchasing more produce, legumes and meats. Your wellness cannot afford the added cost of breakfast cereal, dairy, potato chips, cheese, ice cream, pastries, candy, juices, lunch meat and soda. These items are useless and provide empty calories, which are more expensive than healthier alternatives; omitting them will allow you to have more money for healthier options. A large part of healthy eating and saving money is to avoid processed food and fast food.

"When you shoot for nothing, you will get it every time." - Author Unknown.

While on this journey, focus on your internal motivation, whatever that may be. Our focus, level of our faith and where we spend our energy determines our direction. Distractions come in a variety of forms: friends; past, present or future circumstances; or family members including your spouse. Stay focused on your goals, learn to turn off the negative chatter and tune it out. In martial arts, an idea is taught that will help illustrate this point. When a trained expert stands in front of a stack of bricks he intends to break, he does not focus his attention and energy on the stack itself. Instead, his focus goes beyond the immediate object. He may be focusing on going through the floor, for example. Put your focus where your energy ends. In the same way, when we direct our attention and energy past the result you want, it will carry us through any obstacle until we fully reach the point of focus.

You do not have to go on this journey alone, as I did. I am here to take that ride with you. My goal is for you to build a healthier lifestyle by taking baby steps, looking and feeling your best and building habits that are personalized and permanent. I traveled this road alone for many years not by choice, but because help was not readily available to me. It is now my hope that you will utilize the support that is readily available to you. Take responsibility for what is going on with your health. Ask questions; ask for non-conventional natural health options when possible, versus a conventional approach. The approach shared here is to provide tried-and-true ways to energize, support and strengthen your central nervous system. Holistic treatment can be used in conjunction with conventional medicine to accomplish your goals. Most conventional healthcare professionals are brilliant people and do serve a purpose – but they are not always trained, versed or knowledgeable about natural healthcare practices. I urge you to find a practitioner who will support your journey, goals, values, and beliefs to promote health and wellness.

"Without health, life is not life; it is only a state of languor and suffering - an image of death." - Buddha

Any form of diabetes - whether hypoglycemia, hyperglycemia, type 1 or type 2, or pre-diabetes - is very serious and potentially fatal. Research has shown that these conditions, perhaps with the exception of type 1 diabetes, can be managed or reserved *without* medication, if you participate in a *holistic and healthier lifestyle.* Type 1 diabetics should also consider the benefits of a healthy lifestyle to manage blood sugar levels. This could allow for less aggressive medication types and lower doses of insulin, accordingly. Too little or too much blood sugar (glucose) can be potentially fatal, a battle I have personally fought and won. I shared with you the secrets that have kept me living longer and diabetes free for over 20 years. These are the same secrets and processes I share with my clients; as a result, they too have more energy and stopped feeling guilty about what they eat. They experienced less irritability, rejuvenated skin, lower blood pressure, improved cholesterol level, and stabilized blood sugar. My desire is for you to be healthy; to be drug, pain and disease-free; and to live the life you desire and deserve.

The world we live in today is much different than it was 50 years ago or even 20 years ago. We are continuously exposed to more toxins not just in food, but also in our water, air, clothes, furniture, cookware, toys, cleaning products, building material, medication, and hygiene products. Indeed, some manufacturers have become very creative in how they make and market these products, often using the cheapest means possible; unfortunately, it may be contributing to the declining health crisis in our society. While we may not be able to avoid all chemicals and harmful toxins, we can make a fervent effort to counter many of their effects by the lifestyle we live, for the sake of our well-being.

My beautiful grandmother suffered with pain in her limbs, had her leg amputated and later died in her mid-60s, from complications of diabetes while on medication. I was determined to find a better form of treatment. I was determined to find a way to beat this disease without medication so I could continue to enjoy simple things like bike riding, walks on the beach, and having free mobility of my limbs. I made a decision to create a better lifestyle, all of which was achieved by exploring, discovering and practicing alternative methods.

Keep showing up and taking action. Eventually you will notice the physical, emotional and spiritual transformation. Diabetes, disease, illness, and suffering are NOT your destination. Continue on this journey, and you shall experience improvements and growth every day.

Many Blessings and a Long, Healthy Life!

RECIPES

This is NOT a diet. This is NOT a trend. IT IS A LIFESTYLE CHANGE!

I have included some of my favorite recipes as a sample, to show you that eating healthy can be very passionate and exciting: breakfast, dinner, snacks, side dishes, salad dressing and of course a few special treats. Some of these are Caribbean dishes I learned from my mother and others I have found online. I have made modifications to include some healthier ingredients. Use natural, fresh, and gluten free ingredients when possible. You can alter the ingredient to your liking.

I did not include lunch recipes because I typically eat left over for lunch or eat a brunch. Remember, I plan and pre-cook most of my meals, including most breakfast.

Rule of thumb: It is important to include protein, fats and complex carbs at each meal and snack.

I have chosen these dinner recipes because they have similar ingredients and this is a suggestion of what a weekly meal schedule would look like. How you would plan a weekly meal plan? It looks difficult but once you have the vegetables, herbs and spices ready and season the meats, it is just a matter for cooking.

Simple Tips: Chop all herbs, garlic and onion, in a blender or food processor, and refrigerate for later use.

BREAKFAST

I typically I work out first thing in the morning so usually my breakfast entails a plant based protein shake with a fruit and handful of nuts. I will have one of the following breakfast or brunch items a couple hours later or early noon.

Egg Sandwich
INGREDIENTS

    1-2 eggs poached, scrambled, or fried
    Spray oil
    1-2 slice of sprouted bread (try several brands until you find the one you like)
    Half avocado
    Your choice of meat: grilled chicken; turkey bacon or sausage (optional)
    Small amount of alfalfa sprouts or spinach

DIRECTIONS

    Heat skillet, spray pan and prepare eggs to your liking; lightly toast bread in a toaster, apply egg to read, layer with avocado, meat of choice, and alfalfa sprouts.

Fruit and Nuts Oatmeal
INGREDIENTS

    1-2 cups rolled or steel oats (cook a big pot and reheat when needed)
    Follow cooking directions on package.
    Substitute for water - almond or coconut milk- according to how thick you want it; (any plant or nut based milk)
    ½ tsp. of local honey or coconut nectar (optional)
    ½ cup of choice fruit
    Sprinkle almonds, flaxseeds, or pumpkin seeds before eating

DIRECTIONS

    Follow instruction on the package for the rolled or steel oats. Add fruit last 5 minutes of cooking time. Sprinkle nuts prior to

serving.
Spinach and Spaghetti Squash Quiche
INGREDIENTS
    ½ cup frozen chopped spinach, thawed, and squeezed dry
    ½ cup cooked, shredded spaghetti squash
    1 beaten egg - medium brown, cage free (optional)
    3 egg whites
    1-12 oz. can of coconut milk
    1-cup Daiya shredded mozzarella cheese, dairy-free cheese or fresh mozzarella
    ½ cup rice crumbs

DIRECTIONS

Preheat oven to 400 °F. Slice squash in half, scrape out the seed, place the squash on a roasting pan, and cook for 30-45 minutes depending upon size. It's done when tender, but noodles are a little crunchy. When done, remove from oven and set aside to cool. Reduce oven temperature to 350 °F.

Shred 1/2 cup of squash and place in a mixing bowl. Stir in egg, egg whites, coconut milk, dairy free mozzarella cheese, and spinach until well combined. Spray a 9-inch pie tin or quiche dish with cooking spray. Spread crumbs on the bottom and around the sides to coat. Pour egg mixture into prepared dish. Bake quiche in the preheated oven for 45 minutes, or until a toothpick inserted in the center comes out clean. Allow cooling for at least 10 minutes before cutting. Serve warm or at room temperature.

Portobello Pesto Egg Omelet
INGREDIENTS
    1 tsp. extra virgin olive oil
    1-2 Portobello mushroom caps, slices
    ¼ cup chopped red onions
    2 medium brown eggs (or any egg of your choice)
    ½ tsp. distilled water

Pink Himalayan Sea Salt and ground black pepper to taste
1 tsp. prepared pesto

DIRECTIONS

Heat the olive oil in a skillet over medium heat. Cook the Portobello mushroom and red onion in olive oil until the mushroom has softened, 2 to 3 minutes. In A separate bowl, whisk the eggs, salt and pepper, and water together in a small bowl; pour over the mushroom and onion mixture to coat the small skillet. Cook, until the eggs are no longer runny about five minutes, top with pesto and sprinkle cheese over the mixture. Fold the omelet in half and continue cooking until the cheese melts to your desire, 2 to 3 minutes.

Coconut Flour Waffles

INGREDIENTS:

4 eggs
¼ cup unsalted grass fed butter melted, coconut (liquid form) or olive oil
¼ cup Coconut Flour
1 tbsp. Coconut Flakes (optional)
¼ tsp. Baking Powder
A pinch of Pink Himalayan Sea Salt
2 tbsp. of Coconut Milk (can preferred)

DIRECTIONS:

Heat a waffle maker. Melt butter or coconut oil in a small saucepan over very low heat or double boiler until liquid. In a large bowl, whisk eggs about 1 minute; add melted butter or oil, and milk, whisk together about 1 minute. Add baking powder and salt, whisk for another minute until well blended and no lumps. Fold in coconut flakes. Grease griddle or skillet with oil or butter. Drop ladleful of batter onto hot waffle maker, to cover the area. Cook 3 to 4 minutes or follow the instructions on the maker to determine when it's ready. Serve warm with your favorite pancake toppings. Makes approximately 3 waffles, double the recipe for more.

Fresh Peach and Banana Topping for Waffles, Pancakes, Crepes

INGREDIENTS:
- 1 cup hot water
- 1 tbsp. brown sugar
- 1 tbsp. local honey
- 1 tbsp. arrowroot powder (a little more if you want it thicker)
- Dash of nutmeg
- ¼ tsp. of vanilla extract or essence
- 2 small peaches (leave the skin on) diced
- ½ Banana sliced

DIRECTIONS:

In a small bowl combine water and arrowroot powder until it has blended without lumps. In a large saucepan, combine the water and arrowroot powder mixture, on medium heat, and then add sugar. Bring mixture to a boil while stirring and boil on medium so it does not burn, until the mixture thickens. This should take about 30 seconds to 1 minute. Remove from the heat. Whisk in the nutmeg, extract or essence. Fold in diced peaches and banana until peaches are well coated and combined with the mixture. Serve warm over waffles, pancakes, crepes etc. Makes 4 servings.

MAIN DISH

Caribbean Jerk Chicken

INGREDIENTS:
- 3-4 lbs. of grass-fed or organic chicken breast (bone-in)
- 1 ½ lemon or lime (or 1/4 cup apple cider vinegar)
- 1 cup Walkerswood Jerk Marinade (any jerk seasoning will do)
- 1 tsp. of Walkerswood Hot & Spicy Jerk Seasoning
- ¼ tsp. All Spice
- Pinch of Himalayan pink sea salt and pepper to taste
- ¼ t tsp. pumpkin spice

Salt and pepper to taste

DIRECTIONS:

Wash chicken with ½ lemon or lime. Place chicken in a Ziploc bag. Squeeze one lemon or lime in the bag, add all other ingredients, mix well, and refrigerate for 2-3 hours (overnight is even better). When ready to use, take it out of the refrigerator at least 10 to 20 minutes before. Place meat on a preheat grill or preheat your oven to 375 °F. Place chicken in a baking dish after spraying with it with olive oil (you can also line the pan with aluminum foil for an easier clean up). Bake chicken on the middle rack for 5 minutes, then turn it, leave for another 5 minutes (you don't want to overcook the meat beyond that, because it will be too dry). Then put in the broiler on for another 3- 5 minutes to get a little more color and texture, if needed.

*** This can be eaten with a side of kidney bean and rice or rice pilaf, or mixed steamed vegetables.

Trini Fish Soup

INGREDIENTS:

1 fish head (I used a halibut, red snapper) optional
2 lbs. cubed Cod fish (I use red snapper most times) but use a firm fish
½ large onion chopped
3 scallions
2 tbsp. chopped cilantro
2 tbsp. minced or chopped parsley
1 tbsp. of shado beni or bandanya (found in Asian or West Indian Markets also called cilantro in Asian Markets) optional
1 whole scotch bonnet pepper
3 sprigs thyme
1 tbsp. Worcestershire sauce
2-3 garlic cloves
1 lime (juiced)

8-10 cups water
2 fish stock cubes or any broth or broth base-low sodium
1 tbsp. fish sauce (optional)
¼ tsp. black pepper
1 tbsp. olive oil
1-2 large red potato or sweet potato (cubed)
2-3 green cooking figs
1 carrot
3-4 eddoes also called Taro Root (find in many Asian grocery stores)
1 rib celery
2 cups cubed butternut squash or pumpkin
1-2 cups of chopped spinach
Small bunch watercress (thick stems removed) 3 sprigs thyme

TIP: I like to add a lot of vegetable and root to make it hardy, but you can decide how hardy you want to make it.

DIRECTIONS:

Prepare fish: cut into cubes, make it chunky so it won't shred in the pot; wash with ½ of the lime (reserve the remainder) and drain. You're also using the fish head, make sure you clean the scales and take all the stuff out the middle; add seasoning: black pepper, cilantro, parsley, shado beni, and Worcestershire sauce. Let it marinate for 15-20 minutes. While the fish marinates, get the vegetables ready, once the vegetables are ready. Heat oil in a large stockpot on medium to high heat, add garlic, onion until onion is tender 1-2 minutes. Add celery, and thyme, let cook for 2-3 minutes. Add water, fish cubes or broth; fish sauce, lime, increase heat to high. Add all remaining vegetable and bring to a boil. Reduce heat to medium high cover and boil for 10 minutes; this is the time to do your taste test, add seasoning as needed; add fish, cover and boil for additional 10 minutes. Careful with stirring too much as fish will shred. Taste again and soup should be ready.

TIP: I do not add salt because there is enough salt from the broth or cubes.

Seafood Jambalaya

INGREDIENTS:

1 bag-mixed frozen seafood or you can buy items fresh individually as listed below
1 lb. medium raw shrimp
1 lb. bay scallops
1 lb. calamari
1 lb. mussels
1 lb. fresh crabstick
1 lb. of chicken breast
2-chicken or turkey Italian sausage link
1 tbsp. Worcestershire sauce
2 jalapeno pepper for added spice use 1 jalapeno and 1 habanero
2 large tomatoes
3 scallions
1 large red bell pepper
½ large red onion chopped
2-3 cloves garlic chopped
1 tbsp. chopped cilantro
2 tbsp. minced or chopped parsley
1 tbsp. basil
2-3-rib celery
¼ tsp. black pepper
1 tbsp. creole seasoning (this will give you the salt flavor)
2-3 bay leaves
1 tbsp. olive oil
1 tbsp. raw unsalted grass fed butter (optional)
2 sprigs of thyme
2 tbsp. of oregano
1 tbsp. paprika
3-4 cups of partially cooked brown rice

½ lemon

1-2 tbsp. roux (2 tbsp. unbleached flour and 1 tbsp. olive oil)

DIRECTIONS:

Preheat broiler, place sausage on pan and fully cook. Season chicken with a dash of salt and pepper put in the broiler, for 6 minutes turning half way to not fully cook. Make roux: heat 1 tbsp. oil in a small pan, add 2 tbsp. flour stir continuously until it reaches dark brown but not burnt. (I have tried using coconut flour and other but it does not get the same consistency). Set aside when done. Combine butter and oil in Dutch Oven on medium to high heat, when heated add onion and garlic about 2-3 minutes until onion is tender, add celery, bell pepper, and all herbs and spices, including roux and creole seasoning. Sauté, over medium-high heat for about 8 minutes, or until the natural sugars in the vegetables have browned and caramelized. Add sausage and chicken let cook another 5 minutes. Add the tomatoes and all seafood and bay leaves, and gently stir, add partially cooked rice, stir gently, making sure that the rice is not sticking. Add small amount of water at a time, reduce the heat, cover, and simmer for about 15 minutes or until the rice has absorbed most of the liquid. Turn off the heat, cover, and let sit for about 5 minutes, during which time the jambalaya will continue cooking from residual heat.

Nachos with Ground Turkey

INGREDIENTS:

1 lb. lean ground turkey

2 tbsp. taco seasoning (to taste)

2-3 tbsp. water

2-3 jalapeno pepper

1 large tomato

2 scallions

1 small can of black olive

Chopped cilantro
1 can of vegetarian refried pinto or black beans
1 bag rice chips

DIRECTIONS:

Brown ground turkey in a medium skillet, add taco seasoning and let simmer. If it's too dry add 2-3 tablespoon water. Put the refried beans in a small pot to heat up. Cut vegetables while ground turkey is cooking: When ground turkey is done, serve by placing the chips on a plate add ground turkey, refried bean, add condiments: jalapeno pepper, tomatoes, scallion, black olive, and cilantro in this order. Enjoy!!! You can add cheese and sour cream as a treat if you wish, most times I do not.

Spinach Meat Loaf

INGREDIENTS:
1 ½ - 2 lbs. lean ground turkey
2-3 cups of frozen spinach
16 oz. crushed tomato (you can also crush your own in a blender or food processor)
2 cloves of garlic chopped
1 small onion chopped
1 tbsp. parsley - fresh or dried
1 tbsp. cilantro- fresh or dried
1 tbsp. oregano - fresh or dried
1 tbsp. basil - fresh or dried basil
½ cup of almond, hazelnut or coconut milk
1 tsp. of olive oil
2 large brown eggs
1 tbsp. Italian seasoning
1 tbsp. local honey
1 tbsp. Worcestershire sauce
2 cups rice crumbs
1-2 tsp. dried red crushed chili peppers
Olive Oil Spray
Pinch of Pink Himalayan Sea salt and pepper to taste

2 tbsp. ketchup or 2 tablespoon tomato paste
2 tbsp. barbeque sauce

DIRECTIONS:

Preheat oven to 350 °F. Blend all ingredient except spinach into the ground turkey and mix well; let marinate 15-20 minutes; allow spinach to thaw out: Spray meatloaf pan with pam spray, put half the meatloaf mix into the pan and press firmly to smooth out; layer with spinach, add remaining meatloaf mix and again smooth out with the back of the spoon and press firmly. Place in oven and cook 45 minutes or until fully cook. Cook until center of meatloaf is at least 160 °F.

Chicken and Seafood Pizza

INGREDIENTS:

1 package Garlic and Herb Pizza Dough (Trader Joe's or any brand of your choice)
1 lb. Chicken Breast
1 lb. fresh crab meat or shrimp
1 jar of pesto sauce or Alfredo sauce
1 cup sliced Portobello mushroom
1 red bell pepper- slices
3 cups of fresh or frozen spinach
1 small can sliced black olive
1 cup sliced green zucchini
1 large sliced tomato
5-6 leaves of fresh basil chopped
1 tbsp. red crushed chili pepper (optional)
2 tbsp. coconut flour
Pinch of Pink Himalayan Sea salt, pepper, garlic powder, cayenne pepper to taste

DIRECTIONS:

Preheat oven 450 °F, season chicken with salt, pepper, garlic, cayenne pepper, place in the broiler or sauté on stovetop, cooking only half way and let rest. Follow directions on the dough package to roll out using coconut flour, (roll out to your choice of size and thickness). Place dough on a baking sheet (round or square), add pesto sauce, chicken and crab meat, layer all vegetables, not including black olives or basil; place in the oven for 8-10 minutes, layer black olives and basil put back in for another 2 minutes or until dough is done.

DESSERT

Peach Ice Cream (Dairy-Free Recipe)

You can prepare this delicious dairy free ice cream recipe in less than 5 minutes.

INGREDIENTS:
    1-cup coconut milk (substitute with almond or rice milk)
    1 lb. frozen peach slices (can substitute any fruit of your choosing or use no fruit at all)
    ¼ cup Coconut Crystals (substitute local honey, agave, Stevia) to taste
    ½ tsp. Karibbean Flavours Mixed Essence or vanilla extract
    Pinch of Pink Himalayan Sea salt

DIRECTIONS:

Place all ingredients in blender in the order listed. Follow blender instructions and blend for 30 to 60 seconds.

*** If you do not have a blender, you can also make this in a food processor and put in the freezer for 20 minutes to harden.

Mrs. Parker's Fruit Popsicles (Dairy Free Recipe)
INGREDIENTS:
    2 cups coconut yogurt
    2-3 tbsp. local honey, agave or Stevia (to taste)

1 tsp. Karibbean Flavours Mixed Essence or vanilla extract
3 oz. raspberries
3 oz. of kiwi or strawberries, hulled
6 oz. blueberries
Pinch of Pink Himalayan Sea salt
Optional ingredient: 10 grams of protein powder

DIRECTIONS:

Slice, chop, or lightly blend the fruit to whatever consistency you wish. Combine all ingredients in a bowl and mix well until smooth. Spoon the blueberry mixture evenly between each of the molds. Gently tap the mold on the counter so it levels out. Cover the Popsicle mold with the insert sticks. (If your mold does not come with the stick, you can purchase wooden insert sticks). Place the sticks ¾ of the way into the center of each popsicle. Freeze for four hours or more (overnight is better).

To remove: Set the popsicle mold in a dish of hot water for a moment and gently pull to release the popsicles from the mold. When ready to eat, dip in a small amount of natural granola or sliced almonds. This will be a great alternative breakfast, and the kids will love you.

Gail's Sweet Seduction Treat

INGREDIENTS:

1 cup ground almonds or walnuts
½ cup coconut nectar/agave or rice syrup
½ cup sunflower (or olive, coconut, safflower - any of these will do)
1 cup rolled or steel oat (flaxseed meal also works)
1 ¼ cup spelt or almond flour
½ - 1 jar desired all-fruit preserves (no added sugars)
1 tsp. vanilla extract

DIRECTIONS:
Preheat oven to 350 °F. Mix well, almonds, oats, and flour in a mixing bowl. Stir in all wet ingredients except jam and mix well. Shape into golf-ball size or smaller, and place on a lightly oiled baking sheet. Indent the ball with thumb, fill with all-fruit jam, and close up the ends. Bake for approximately 15 to 20 minutes.

Awesome Cupcake

INGREDIENTS:

2 cups coconut flour (optional: if you want it more fluffy, lighter, 2 cups cake flour will produce a lighter cupcake than all-purpose)

2 tsp. baking powder

1 tsp. sea salt

6 tbsp. (1 stick) unsalted, grass fed butter at room temperature

4 tbsp. olive oil or coconut oil

1 cup coconut sugar

1 tbsp. vanilla extract reserved

2 large egg whites, at room temperature

2 large whole eggs, at room temperature

¾ cup coconut milk, at room temperature

Oil Spray

Optional Topping:

1½ cup canned coconut milk refrigerated

4 tsp. powdered sugar

1 tsp. vanilla flavoring or vanilla extract

1 pint strawberries, washed, hulled and sliced

1 pint blueberries, washed

DIRECTIONS:

Preheat the oven to 350 °F. Place one rack in the middle. Line two pans of 1-dozen-each muffin tins (1 cup size) with paper liners or grease well with pam spray. In a medium bowl, combine the dry ingredients (flour, baking powder and salt) and mix well to break up any lumps. Set aside. Place butter in the bowl; use beater, or stand mixer and beat on medium-high speed until very light in color, about 3 minutes. Add sugar and continue beating until it is light and airy, about 3 minutes. Scrape down the paddle and the sides of the bowl. Turn the mixer to medium speed and, one at a time, add the egg whites, beating well to incorporate after each addition. Then add the eggs one at a time, again beating well after each addition. Add the milk, add the vanilla extract here, and mix until combined. It will look lumpy. Scrape down the sides of the bowl. Reduce the speed to low, add the mixed dry ingredients and fold together until just combined, about 15-30 seconds.

Fill the muffin tin each about halfway (3-4 ounces each). If a well or two does not get filled, fill it with ½ cup water instead. Bake in preheated oven until the cupcakes are golden brown on top and a toothpick inserted into the center comes out clean, roughly 14 to 16 minutes. Set the pans on a wire rack and let cool for 5 minutes. Remove the cupcakes from the pans and let cool completely before topping.

While the cupcakes are cooling, put the cream in a mixing bowl with a wire whip attachment (or whip by hand with a whisk). Stir in the sugar and vanilla, then whip to stiff peaks, but not dry.

Immediately before serving, top cooled cupcakes with a dollop of coconut whipped cream and fruit.

SIDE DISHES

Spicy Sweet Potato Oven Fries
INGREDIENTS:
- 1.5 to 2 lbs. sweet potatoes (partially or totally peeled)
- 1½ tbsp. olive oil

1 tsp. Italian seasoning

1 tsp. of rosemary

1 tsp. smoked paprika

¼ tsp. cayenne pepper (to taste)

Pinch of cinnamon or pumpkin spice

½ tsp. Pink Himalayan Sea salt (to taste)

½ tsp. black pepper

DIRECTIONS:

Preheat oven to 350 °F. Coat two baking sheets with cooking spray or cover with parchment paper. Cut sweet potatoes into ½ inch shoestring strips and place in a large bowl. Add all dry ingredients in a small bowl and mix well. Drizzle olive oil over potatoes. Toss vigorously to coat. Add dry ingredients from the small bowl and toss until evenly distributed. Spread potatoes out on prepared baking sheets so the pieces are not touching. (If placed too close they will sweat and become too moist). Place in preheated oven and bake for 20 to 25 minutes. Increase the oven temperature to 425 °F. Using a spatula, toss or turn over the fries on the baking sheet, and bake for 10 to 15 more minutes or until the potato exterior is lightly browned and blistered. Remove from oven, season with additional salt to taste if needed, and serve.

SNACK

Spicy Hummus

INGREDIENTS:

1 can or 14.5 ounce cooked chickpeas/garbanzo beans drained (save the reserves)

2 tbsp. tahini sesame paste

A drizzle extra-virgin olive oil

½ teaspoon crushed pepper flakes

½-1 jalapeno pepper

1 tsp. (1/3 palm full) ground cumin

1 tsp. (1/3 palm full) ground coriander
1-2 clove garlic
Coarse Sea Salt
½ lemon, juiced
Serve with pita breads, grilled and cut into wedges for dipping, celery stick, broccoli or rice crackers

DIRECTIONS:
Combine beans, tahini, oil, pepper flakes, cumin, coriander, garlic, salt, and lemon juice in food processor bowl or blender and grind into a smooth paste. If it's too thick add small drops of the reserves until smooth paste is reach. Transfer to a small dip dish and surround spread with warm pita wedges or other options above.

P, B, & J
INGREDIENTS:
Almond, cashew or peanut butter
Natural fruit preserves (read the label or added sugar)
1-2 slices - sprout or whole grain bread

Apple with Almond Butter
INGREDIENTS:
1-2 tbsp. almond, peanut or cashew butter
1 small apple sliced
You can also use almond butter, with prunes, celery, broccoli or rice crackers

HOMEMADE SALAD DRESSING

White wine Dijon
3 tbsp. Dijon mustard
3 tbsp. dry white wine
1 tsp. rosemary
½ tsp, kosher sea salt, and white pepper to taste.

Gradually whisk in ½-cup olive oil or walnut oil
Allow marinating 2-4 hrs. (overnight is better)

Lemon Mustard

Whisk 2 tbsp. lemon or lime juice
1 tbsp. Dijon mustard
1 tsp. lemon zest
½ tsp. coconut sugar or honey
Salt to taste
Gradually whisk in ¼ cup each of olive oil and walnut or grapeseed oil.
Allow marinating 2-4 hrs. (overnight is better)

Red Orange-Walnut

Whisk 2 tbsp. orange juice
1 tsp. sherry brandy or dry red wine
1 tsp. apple cider vinegar
½ tsp. sea salt and white pepper to taste.
Gradually whisk in 3 tablespoons each walnut oil and olive oil.
Allow marinating 2-4 hrs. (overnight is better)

BIBLIOGRAPHY

Academy of Health Science Curriculum. Carb Loading. http://www.thehealthscienceacademy.org

Adams, M. Health Ranger Habits & Avoid List. *Natural Health Is Our DNA - EnCogitive.com.* http://www.encognitive.com/node/7097.

American Diabetes Association. Hyperglycemia (High Blood Glucose) - What causes hyperglycemia, September 16, 2014. http://www.diabetes.org/living-with-diabetes/treatment-and-care/blood-glucose-control/hyperglycemia.html.

American Heart Association. Sugar 101. Accessed May 1, 2017. http://www.heart.org/ HEARTORG/GettingHealthy/NutritionCenter/HealthyEating/Sugar101_UCM_306024_Article.jsp.

Amiel, S.A., Dixon, T., Mann, R. and Jameson, K. Hypoglycaemia in Type 2 diabetes: *Diabet Med. 25(3): Mar , 2008;245–254.doi:* 10.1111/j.1464-5491.2007.02341.x*: PMCID: PMC2327221.* Retrieved from http://www.ncbi.nlm.nih.gov/pmc/articles/PMC2327221/.

Arthritis Foundation. 8 Food Ingredients That Can Cause Inflammation. Accessed January 14, 2017. http://www.arthritis.org/living-with-arthritis/arthritis-diet/foods-to-avoid-limit/food-ingredients-and-inflammation-11.php.

Avena, N.M., Rada P., Hoebel B.G. Evidence For Sugar Addiction: Behavioral and Neurochemical Effects of Intermittent, Excessive Sugar Intake. Neurosci Biobehav Rev. *2008;32(1):20-39.* Epub 2007 May 18. http://www.ncbi.nlm.nih.gov/pubmed/17617461.

Bagozzi, D. WHO Launches The First Global Strategy on Traditional and Alternative Medicine. *World Health Organization*, May 20, 2002. http://www.who.int/mediacentre/news/releases/release38/en/.

Beaglehole, R. and Lefèbvre, P. Diabetes Action Now – An Initiative of the World Health Organization and the International Diabetes Federation 2004. http://www.who.int/diabetes/actionnow/en/DANbooklet.pdf, pg 4, 15.

Beattie, D. What Percentage Of New Gym Members In January Stop Coming After February? January 2012. https://www.quora.com/What-percentage-of-new-gym-members-in-January-stop-coming-after-February.

Bobalik, J. How to Calculate Your Training Heart Rate Zones. http://www.active.com/fitness/articles/how-to-calculate-your-training-heart-rate-zones?page=2.

Broadfoot, M.V Why Do Our Bodies Make Icky Mucus. *The News & Observer, May 30, 2011.* http://www.newsobserver.com/news/technology/article23721178.html.

Breene, S. Why The Snooze Button Is Ruining Your Sleep, October 14, 2014. http://greatist.com/happiness/snooze-button-bad-for-sleep.

Bryce, M. Artificial Dyes In The Foods We Consume And Feed To Our Children: Health Effects by Color. Retrieved from http://www.whydye.org/resources/health-effects-by-color/.

Cann, K. Type 3 Diabetes, The Next Epidemic? http://robbwolf.com/2015/03/25/type-3-diabetes-the-next-epidemic/.

Carey, E. 10 Processed Foods to Avoid, September 19, 2014. http://www.healthline.com/health/food-nutrition/processed-foods-to-avoid.

Chang, K. Artificial Sweeteners May Disrupt Body's Blood Sugar Controls. *New York Times Blog,* September 14, 2014. http://well.blogs.nytimes.com/2014/09/17/artificial-sweeteners-may-disrupt-bodys-blood-sugar-controls/?_r=0.

Cheren, M., Foushi , M., Gudmundsdotter, E. H., Hillcock, C., Lerner, M., Prager, M., Rice, M., Walsh, L., Werdell, P. Physical Craving and Food Addiction: A Scientific Review. A Scientific Paper, 2009. Retrieved from http://foodaddictioninstitute.org/scientific-research/physical-craving-and-food-addiction-a-scientific-review/.

Cleveland Clinic. Digestive System - Diseases & Conditions. Cleveland Clinic. Accessed March 23, 2017. http://my.clevelandclinic.org/health/diseases_conditions/hic_The_Structure_and_Function_of_the_Digestive_System, 1995-2017.

Crunchy Betty. 21 Things You Should Know About Using Essential Oils, February 23, 2017. http://www.crunchybetty.com/21-things-you-should-know-about-essential-oils.

Daily Intake Guide – Australian Food and Grocery Council. Accessed February 9, 2017. http://www.mydailyintake.net/nutrients/.

DiNicolantonio, J. J. and Lucan, S. Sugar Season. It's Everywhere, and Addictive, December 22, 2014. *New York Times*. https://www.nytimes.com/2014/12/23/opinion/sugar-season-its-everywhere-and-addictive.html.

Dowshen, S. Childhood Stress. *The Kids Health Organization*, February 2015. http://kidshealth.org/parent/emotions/feelings/stress.html.

Fowler, S.P., Williams, K., Resendez R.G., Hunt K. J., Hazuda H.P. and Stern M.P. Fueling the Obesity Epidemic? Artificially Sweetened Beverage Use and Long-term Weight Gain, August 2008. DOI: 10.1038/oby.2008.284: http://onlinelibrary.wiley.com/doi/10.1038/oby.2008.284/abstract.

Gavura, S. Food Allergies: Facts, Myths, and Pseudoscience. Science Based Medicine, September 12, 2013. https://www.sciencebasedmedicine.org/food-allergies-facts-myths-and-pseudoscience/.

Gene Smart. List of Aerobic Exercises. Accessed November 28, 2016. http://www.genesmart.com/pages/aerobic_activity/89.php.

Glycemic Edge. Glycemic Index Diet & Diabetes Health. Accessed April 8, 2017. http://www.glycemicedge.com/glycemic-index-chart/.

Gray, L. Will Today's Children Die Earlier Than Their Parents. *BBC News Magazine*, July 8, 2014. http://www.bbc.com/news/magazine-28191865.

Gunnars, K. Is Dairy Bad For You, or Good? The Milky, Cheesy Truth. http://authoritynutrition.com/is-dairy-bad-or-good/.

Halpin, H.A., Suárez-Varela, M.M., Martin-Moreno, J. Chronic Disease Prevention and the New Public Health, June 2010. http://www.publichealthreviews.eu/show/f/24.

Harvard Medical School. Sleep, Performance, and Public Safety, December 8, 2007. Accessed May 5, 2017. http://healthysleep.med.harvard.edu/healthy/matters/consequences/sleep-performance-and-public-safety.

Harvard Medical School, Patient Education Center. Sinusitis: Inflammation and infection. Accessed December 11, 2016. http://www.patienteducationcenter.org/articles/sinusitis-inflammation-and-infection/.

Harvard School of Public Health. Obesity Prevention Source - Sleep. Accessed February 13, 2017. http://www.hsph.harvard.edu/obesity-prevention-source/obesity-causes/sleep-and-obesity/.

Hunsinger B., D. Mom Has Biggest Impact on Girls' Body Image, August 23, 2013. http://www.usatoday.com/story/news/nation/2013/08/23/moms-daughters-influence-body-image/2690921/.

Hyman, M. How Eating at Home Can Save Your Life, January 9, 2011. http://www.huffingtonpost.com/dr-mark-hyman/family-dinner-how_b_806114.html.

Isaacson, B. Our Sleep Problem and What to Do About It, January 22, 2015. http://www.newsweek.com/2015/01/30/our-sleep-problem-and-what-do-about-it-301165.html.

Ismail-Beigi, F. Glycemic Management of Type 2 Diabetes Mellitus. 366:1319-1327, April 5, 2012. DOI: 10.1056/NEJMcp1013127. http://www.nejm.org/doi/full/10.1056/NEJMcp1013127.

Johns Hopkins Bloomberg School of Public Health. Home Cooking is a Main Ingredient in Healthier Diet, November 17, 2014. Accessed March, 22, 2017. http://www.jhsph.edu/research/centers-and-institutes/johns-hopkins-center-for-a-livable-future/news-room/News-Releases/2014/Study-Suggests-Home-Cooking-Main-Ingredient-in-Healthier-Diet.html.

Johns Hopkins Medicine. Research Involving Food or Food-Derived Products, Spices/Herbs, or Dietary Supplements, April 2012. Accessed September 9, 2016. http://www.hopkinsmedicine.org/institutional_review_board/guidelines_policies/guidelines/ind_not_drugs.html

Kearney, J. Food Consumption Trends And Drivers. *Dublin Institute of Technology, Vol. 365, No. 1554*, pp. 2793-2807, August 16, 2010. http://rstb.royalsocietypublishing.org/content/royptb/365/1554/2793.full.pdf.

Krantz, R. 7 Reasons Milk is Bad for you, January 25, 2016. http://www.bustle.com/articles/137195-7-reasons-milk-is-bad-for-you.

Kravitz, L. Exercise Motivation: What Starts and Keeps People Exercising? *Johnson Health Tech North America Inc. https://www.unm.edu/~lkravitz/Article%20folder/ExerciseMot.pdf.*

LA Fitness. Does Our Body Process Artificial Sweeteners The Same As Regular Sugar? April 3, 2014. Accessed October 15, 2016. http://blog.lafitness.com/2014/04/03/does-our-body-process-artificial-sweeteners-the-same-as-regular-sugar/.

Lally, P., van Jaarsveld, C., Potts, H.W.W., Wardle, J. How Are Habits Formed: Modelling Habit Formation In The Real World. *European Journal of Social Psychology*, July 16, 2009. DOI: 10.1002/ejsp.674. http://onlinelibrary.wiley.com/doi/10.1002/ejsp.674/abstract;jsessionid=0DD082A31ECD0532B72794707701053E.f02t01.

Laskow, S. Americans Spend Twice As Much Of Our Budgets On Processed Food As We Did 30 Years Ago, June 13, 2012. http://grist.org/food/americans-spend-twice-as-much-of-our-budgets-on-processed-food-as-we-did-30-years-ago/

Life Extension. Inflammation (Chronic). Accessed May 8, 2017. http://www.lifeextension.com/Protocols/Health-Concerns/Chronic-Inflammation/Page-01.

Lindenmuth, K. The 6 Veggies with the Most Protein. *Women's Health*, March 13, 2014. http://www.womenshealthmag.com/nutrition/high-protein-vegetables.

Main, E. Hidden Dangers Of Artificial Sweeteners. Convinced Going No-cal Is A Good Way To Get Your Sugar Fix? Think Again, May 18, 2015. http://www.rodalesorganiclife.com/food/dangers-artificial-sweeteners.

Maltby, J., Lewis, C.A. and Day, L. Prayer And Subjective Well-being: The Application of A Cognitive-behavioural Framework. *Mental Health Religion and Culture, Sheffield Hallam University Research Archive (SHURA) 2008, 11 (1), 119-129.* http://shura.shu.ac.uk/6056/1/Day_Prayer_and.pdf.

Marcelle, P. Type 3 Diabetes. Women Transforming Women's Health for over 30 years. https://www.womentowomen.com/insulin-resistance/type-3-diabetes/.

Martin, T., Campbell, K. R. Vitamin D and Diabetes. *American Diabetes Association. May; 24(2): 113-118.* http://spectrum.diabetesjournals.org/content/24/2/113.full.

Massachusetts Medical Society. Reduction In The Incidence of Type 2 Diabetes With Lifestyle Intervention or Metformin. *Diabetes Prevention Program Research Group, February 7, 2002 No. 6,* http://www.nejm.org/doi/pdf/10.1056/NEJMoa012512.

Massachusetts Medical Society. The Effects of Intensive Treatment of Diabetes on the Development and Progression of Long-Term Complications in Insulin-Dependent Diabetes Mellitus. *The Diabetes Control and Complications Trial Research Center: September 30, 1993, No.14, 329:977-986, DOI: 10.1056/NEJM199309303 291401.* http://www.nejm.org/doi/full/10.1056/NEJM199309303291401.

Mayo Clinic Staff. Chronic Stress Puts Your Health at Risk: Chronic Stress Can Wreak Havoc on Your Mind and Body, April 21, 2016. Accessed December 14, 2016. http://www.mayoclinic.

org/healthy-lifestyle/stress-management/in-depth/stress/art-20046037.

May Clinic Staff. Red Wine and Resveratrol: Good For Your Heart. Accessed May 2, 2017. http://www.mayoclinic.org/diseases-conditions/heart-disease/in-depth/red-wine/art-20048281.

Mercola, J. Artificial Sweeteners - More Dangerous Than You Ever Imagined, October 13, 2009. http://articles.mercola.com/sites/articles/archive/2009/10/13/artificial-sweeteners-more-dangerous-than-you-ever-imagined.aspx.

Mercola, J. Doctor Says: If There's a Single Marker Lifespan, This Would Be Insulin Sensitivity. June 6, 2012. http://articles.mercola.com/sites/articles/archive/2012/06/06/eft-on-chronic-inflammation.aspx.

Mercola, J. First Case Study to Show Direct Link Between Alzheimer's and Aluminum Toxicity, March 22, 2014. http://articles.mercola.com/sites/articles/archive/2014/03/22/aluminum-toxicity-alzheimers.aspx.

Mercola, J. Why You Should Avoid Frozen Foods, April 11, 2006. http://articles.mercola.com/sites/articles/archive/2006/04/11/stay-away-from-frozen-foods.aspx.

More Jolts. Time Elapsed. Accessed April 10, 2017. http://www.wiley.com/legacy/email_templates/Thiagi_More_Jolts.pdf

My Body Tutor. Why Does Eating Every 3-4 Hours Work? Accessed February 16, 2017. http://www.mybodytutor.com/pages/eating-every-3-4-hours.

Nathan, D.M., Buse, J.B., Davidson M.B., Ferrannini, E., Holman, R.R., Sherwin, R., and Zinman, B. Medical Management of Hyperglycemia in Type 2 Diabetes: A Consensus Algorithm for the Initiation and Adjustment of Therapy, 32(1) Jan 2009; 193–203. doi: *10.2337/dc08-9025*: PMCID: PMC2606813. https://doi.org/10.2337/dc08-9025.

National Diabetes Statistics Report, 2014. Accessed March 30, 2017. http://www.cdc.gov/diabetes/pubs/statsreport14/national-diabetes-report-web.pdf.

National Health Services Choices. Eating Processed Foods, January 6, 2017. Accessed May 6, 2017. http://www.nhs.uk/livewell/goodfood/pages/what-are-processed-foods.aspx.

National Institutes of Health and the Friends of the National Library of Medicine. The
Mind Body Connection, Winter 2008 Issue: Vol 3 No. 1. Accessed March 17, 2017. https://medlineplus.gov/magazine/issues/winter08/articles/winter08pg4.html.

National Sleep Foundation. How Much Sleep Do We Really Need. Accessed April 29, 2017. http://sleepfoundation.org/how-sleep-works/how-much-sleep-do-we-really-need.

Noel, Rose. All About Autoimmunity. *Irish American, August/September 2013*. http://irishamerica.com/2013/08/all-about-autoimmunity-ask-the-expert-dr-noel-rose/.

Papini, S.C., Pugliese, M.A, Calaudia, A., Gershwin, M.E. Environmental Pathways to Autoimmune Diseases: the Cases of Primary Biliary Cirrhosis and Multiple Sclerosis. *Arch Med Sci. 2011 Jun; 7(3): 368–380*. Published online 2011 Jul 11. doi: 10.5114/aoms.2011.23398 PMCID: PMC3258751. https://www.ncbi.nlm.nih.gov/pubmed/22295019.

Petrovska, B.B. Historical Review of Medicinal Plants' Usage, 2012 Jan-Jun; 6(11): 1–5. http://www.ncbi.nlm.nih.gov/pmc/articles/PMC3358962/.

Phlegm. 2017. Merriam-Webster. Retrieved May 20, 2017 from https://www.merriam-webster.com/dictionary/phlegm.

Potts, J., Carnegie Mellon Today: Carnegie Mellon, University of Pittsburgh Scientists Discover Biological Basis for Autism. http://www.cmu.edu/cmnews/extra/040809_autism.html.

Reader's Digest. 4 Most Harmful Ingredients in Packaged Foods. Accessed March 31, 2017 http://www.rd.com/health/diet-weight-loss/4-most-harmful-ingredients-in-packaged-foods/3/#ixzz3SytX5NjF.

Seaberg, M. Can Meditation Cure Disease? December 25, 2010. http://www.thedailybeast.com/articles/2010/12/25/can-meditation-cure-disease.html.

Selmi, C., Papini, A.M., Pugliese, P., Alcaro, M.C., and Gershwin, M. E. Environmental Pathways to Autoimmune Diseases: The Cases of Primary Biliary Cirrhosis and Multiple Sclerosis. http://www.ncbi.nlm.nih.gov/pmc/articles/PMC3258751/.

Scott, C. Misconceptions About Aerobic and Anaerobic Energy Expenditure. *Journal of the International Society of Sports Nutrition 2.2 (2005): 32. BioMed Central.* https://www.ncbi.nlm.nih.gov/pmc/articles/PMC2129144/.

Sharma, A., Madaan, V., *Petty*, F.D. Exercise for Mental Health. *The Primary Care Companion 2006; 8(2): 106.* http://www.ncbi.nlm.nih.gov/pmc/articles/PMC1470658/.

Society for Cardiovascular Angiography and Interventions. Meditation &Your Heart: Stress-Buster May Reduce Risk for Heart Attack & Stroke, September 11, 2014. Accessed May 19, 2017. http://www.scai.org/image.axd?id=440291a3-244e-4a8c-8ec9-b0857b414d94.

Spiritual Now. The Different Types of Meditation, October 20, 2006. Accessed March 21, 2017 http://www.spiritualnow.com/articles/20/1/The-Different-Types-of-Meditation/Page1.html

Stojanovich L., Marisavljevich D. Stress As A Trigger of Autoimmune Disease. Autoimmun Rev. 2008 Jan;7(3):209-13. doi: 10.1016/j.autrev.2007.11.007. Epub 2007 Nov 29. http://www.ncbi.nlm.nih.gov/pubmed/18190880.

Swanson, A. Big Pharmaceutical Companies Are Spending Far More On Marketing Than Research. *The Washington Post, February 11,2015.* https://www.washingtonpost.com/news/wonk/wp/2015/02/11/big-pharmaceutical-companies-are-spending-far-more-on-marketing-than-research/.

Thompson, J. Strength and Cardio Training: Should They Mix? July 28, 2014. Accessed October 3, 2016. https://www.johnsonfit.com/blog/strength-and-cardio-training-should-they-mix.

United States Department of Agriculture, June 10, 2015. Accessed July 17, 2016. http://www.choosemyplate.gov/physical-activity/why.html.

United States Department of Health and Human Services. Symptoms & Causes of Diabetes. Accessed November 12, 2016. http://www.niddk.nih.gov/health-information/health-topics/Diabetes/causes-diabetes/Pages/index.aspx.

University of Maryland Medical Center. Diabetes. Accessed January 8, 2017. https://umm.edu/health/medical/altmed/condition/diabetes.

University of Maryland Medical Center. Herbal Medicine: Accessed March 11, 2017. http://umm.edu/health/medical/altmed/treatment/herbal-medicine.

University of Maryland Medical Center. Stress, January 30, 2013. Accessed March 27, 2017. http://umm.edu/health/medical/reports/articles/stress.

U.S. Department of Health and Human Services. What happened to the President's Challenge? Accessed May 8, 2017. https://www.presidentschallenge.org/motivated/strengthening.html.

U.S. Food & Drug Administration. Are Dietary Supplements Approved By FDA? March 4, 2014. Accessed February 25, 2017. http://www.fda.gov/AboutFDA/Transparency/Basics/ucm194344.htm.

U.S. Food & Drug Administration. Dietary Supplements. April 14, 2017. https://www.fda.gov/forconsumers/consumerupdates/ucm153239.html.

U.S. Food & Drug Administration. Fortify Your Knowledge About Vitamins, September 20, 2016. Accessed March 13, 2017. http://www.fda.gov/ForConsumers/ConsumerUpdates/ucm118079.html.

U.S. Food & Drug Administration. Regulatory Guidance Drug Registration and Listing, December 9, 2014. Accessed May 19, 2017. https://www.fda.gov/Drugs/GuidanceCompliance RegulatoryInformation/DrugRegistrationandListing/ucm084014.htm.

U.S. National Library of Medicine. Vitamins. Accessed September 25, 2016 https://www.nlm.nih.gov/medlineplus/ency/

article/002399.html.

VoL.T. What America Spends On Groceries. Planet Money-The Economy Explained. http://www.npr.org/sections/money/2012/06/08/154568945/what-america-spends-on-groceries.

Wallace, M. The Digestive System & How it Works, September 2013. http://www.niddk.nih.gov/health-information/health-topics/Anatomy/your-digestive-system/Pages/anatomy.aspx.

Wallace, R. The Importance of Exercise & Nutrition, Jul 04, 2015. Accessed June 29, 2016. http://www.livestrong.com/article/451983-the-importance-of-exercise-nutrition/.

Wehrwein, P. Astounding Increase in Antidepressant Use by Americans. *Harvard Health Publications - Harvard Medical School, October 20, 2011.* http://www.health.harvard.edu/blog/astounding-increase-in-antidepressant-use-by-americans-201110203624.

Wexler, S.Z. Exercise Vs. Diet: The Truth About Weight Loss. *Huffpost, April 30, 2014.* http://www.huffingtonpost.com/2014/04/30/exercise-vs-diet-for-weightloss_n_5207271.html.

Willingham, V. Reversing Diabetes is Possible. http://www.cnn.com/2011/HEALTH/01/28/reverse.diabetes.

World's Healthiest Foods. What Are the Problems With Processed Food? May 2017. Accessed May 16, 2017. http://www.whfoods.com/genpage.php?tname=george&dbid=107.

World's Healthiest Foods. What is the Glycemic Index? May 2017. Accessed May 16, 2017. The World's Healthiest Foods. Whfoods.org. May 2017. http://tinyurl.com/ntw9q9q.

Zamora, D. and Nazario, B. New Year's Resolution: Get Fit, November 30, 2007. http://www.webmd.com/fitness-exercise/new-years-resolution-get-fit.

Zinczenko, D. Noll, E. and Metz, J. Real Money: Fast Food Versus Home-Cooked Meals. *ABC NEWS via WORLD NEWS, January 22, 2014.* http://abcnews.go.com/blogs/lifestyle/2014/01/real-money-fast-food-versus-home-cooked-meals/.

Made in the USA
Lexington, KY
18 April 2018